The Complete Guide to CBD Hemp Oil

Cure Anxiety, Relief Pain, And Improve Health.

Jason Grant

Contents

INTRODUCTION

CHAPTER ONE

Cannabidiol (CBD) Uses for Pain, Inflammation, Epilepsy & More

CBD Hemp Oil – A Natural Way to Perfect Health

CBD Oil for Anxiety: Treating Anxiety Disorders Safely

Benefits of CBD Oil (Cannabidiol) & Why It's Not What You Think.

How Can You Treat Anxiety with Cannabis Oil?

CHAPTER TWO

Healing with Hemp Oil: Your Ultimate Guide to CBD Oil

Hemp and Inflammation Pain Relief

CBD Oil and Arthritis Pain Relief

CBD Oil for Pain Management: Natural, Safe Pain Relief that Actually Works

CHAPTER THREE

Hemp-based Alternative Pain Treatments

4 Ways CBD Oil Can Help Improve Your Life

CBD Hemp Oil Helpful in Daily Life?

7 Observations from Using Hemp Oil Every Day for Three Months

Does CBD Hemp Oil Have Side Effects?

CBD Hemp Oil and Animals

CONCLUSION

INTRODUCTION

CBD oil, also known as hemp oil, is derived from the cannabis plant. Unlike the cannabis that you see people smoke, CBD oil is free from (or has extremely low levels of) THC (tetrahydrocannabinol). This is the chemical that causes cannabis users to feel 'high'. CBD (short for cannabidiol) is another cannabis-derived chemical. While also offering numerous therapeutic effects, it does not induce a 'high' or have any intoxicating effects. One of the most potent therapeutic effects of CBD is its anti-anxiety properties. Cannabidiol, or CBD, is extracted from hemp or cannabis plants. Cannabidiol is one of over 60 compounds called cannabinoids. These are found in a variety of plants, but the most well-known are those found in cannabis. If you haven't heard of CBD oil and its health benefits before, read on to discover just what CBD oil is and how it can help you deal with your anxiety. CBD pain relief works by interacting with the endocannabinoid receptors in your brain and immune system. CBD oil claims many benefits that seem to include every imaginable ailment. It's a good idea to look a little deeper whenever something seems to be a cure-all.

CHAPTER ONE

Cannabidiol (CBD) Uses for Pain, Inflammation, Epilepsy & More

People take or apply cannabidiol to treat a variety of symptoms, but its use is controversial. There is some confusion about what it is and the effects it has on the human body.

Cannabidiol (CBD) may have some health benefits, and it may also pose risks. Products containing the compound are now legal in many American states where marijuana is not.

What is CBD oil?

CBD is one of many compounds, known as cannabinoids, in the cannabis plant. Researchers have been looking at the potential therapeutic uses of CBD.

Oils that contain concentrations of CBD are known as CBD oils. The concentrations and the uses of these oils vary.

Is CBD marijuana?

Until recently, the best-known compound in cannabis was delta-9 tetrahydrocannabinol (THC). This is the most active ingredient in marijuana.

Marijuana contains both THC and CBD, and these compounds have different effects.

THC creates a mind-altering "high" when it is broken down by heat and introduced into the body. This results from smoking marijuana or using it in cooking, for example.

Unlike THC, CBD is not psychoactive. This means that it does not change the state of mind of the person who uses it.

However, CBD does appear to produce significant changes in the body, and some research suggests that it has medical benefits.

The least processed form of the cannabis plant, known as hemp, contains most of the CBD used medicinally. Though hemp and marijuana come from the same plant, Cannabis sativa, the two are very different.

Over the years, marijuana farmers have selectively bred their plants to contain high levels of THC and other compounds that interested them, often because the compounds produced a smell or had another effect on the plant's flowers.

However, hemp farmers have rarely modified the plant. These hemp plants are used to create CBD oil.

How CBD works

All cannabinoids, including CBD, produce effects in the body by attaching to certain receptors.

The human body produces certain cannabinoids on its own. It also has two receptors for cannabinoids, called the CB1 receptors and CB2 receptors.

CB1 receptors are located throughout the body, but many are in the brain.

The CB1 receptors in the brain deal with coordination and movement, pain, emotions, and mood, thinking, appetite, and memories, among other factors. THC attaches to these receptors.

CB2 receptors are more common in the immune system. They affect inflammation and pain.

Researchers once believed that CBD attached to these CB2 receptors, but it now appears that CBD does not attach directly to either receptor. Instead, it seems to direct the body to use more of its own cannabinoids.

What is CBD hemp oil?

CBD is an abbreviation for "cannabidiol" - one of over 113 phytocannabinoids that are naturally occurring in cannabis. CBD by itself has no psychoactive effects (no marijuana 'high' because it is NOT marijuana/THC). CBD, as well as other cannabinoids, have been shown to have properties, when ingested or applied topically, that may benefit your health. Cannabinoids like CBD can be found in hemp, and our proprietary genetics, biodynamic farming practices, and supercritical CO_2 extraction process create the most pure and most potent product on the market.

Cannabinoid Research Has Shown Potential Positive Effects for a Range of Issues!

You can search the National Institutes of Health or Google Scholar to find research for cannabinoids like CBD!

The Endocannabinoid System in You

You have an "endocannabinoid system" in your body. Every human does! This is one of science's most exciting discoveries - each of us are basically "pre-wired" with cannabinoid receptors throughout our body! These receptors are most abundant in our immune system and in our brain - two extremely important functions for optimal health and wellness.

Can CBD Hemp Oil help me?

Due to federal regulations, no claims can be made about any specific ailments that may be alleviated or cured with the use of CBD

Hemp Oil. However, you can do your own research with the product and see if it helps you.

CBD oil is a great remedy for a lot of different ailments. Here are some of the amazing uses people (and medical research) report for CBD oil:

1. Relief for Chronic Pain

Those suffering from chronic pain from diseases like fibromyalgia are finding relief with CBD. Taking CBD can offer pain relief and can even prevent nervous system degeneration. In fact, it has been approved in Canada for multiple sclerosis and cancer pain.

What's really amazing is that CBD doesn't cause dependence or tolerance, so it's a great choice for those trying to stay away from opioids.

Other Remedies to Consider: Not into CBD? Research also shows that turmeric consumption and heat therapy (like sauna use) may be helpful as well. A low inflammation diet also seems to be helpful for some people.

2. Calms Childhood Epilepsy

CBD has anti-seizure properties that have been shown to successfully treat drug-resistant children who have neurological disorders like epilepsy (with no side effects!).

Other Remedies to Consider: Childhood epilepsy is a serious condition and it is important to work with a qualified practitioner with a specialty in this area. Emerging research also shows that a ketogenic diet can be very helpful for drug resistant epilepsy, especially in children.

3. Reduces Anxiety and Depression

According to the Anxiety and Depression Association of America, depression affects 6% and anxiety affects 18% of the U.S. population each year. Research shows that CBD oil can help with both.

CBD has been shown to reduce levels of stress and anxiety in those suffering from conditions such as PTSD, social anxiety disorder, and obsessive compulsive disorder. CBD even reduced the stress and discomfort surrounding public speaking.

Though a B12 deficiency may also be to blame, CBD has been shown to reduce depression by enhancing both serotonergic and glutamate cortical signaling (both are lacking in those with depression).

Other Remedies to Consider: Vitamin B12 is also linked to mental health and it may be helpful to work with someone experienced in optimizing levels of B12.

4. Fights Multi-Drug Resistant Bacteria

Researchers discovered that cannabinoids (including CBD) have an unusual ability to destroy bacteria (especially drug-resistant strains). More research is needed to find out how and why it works.

Whatever the mechanism is for destroying bacteria, CBD seems to be a potent weapon against the antibiotic resistant "superbugs" that are becoming more and more of a problem today.

Other Remedies to Consider: Don't want to try cannabidiol? There is also research on using garlic, honey and oregano oil for drug resistant strains, but work with a practitioner experienced in infectious disease.

5. Reduces Inflammation

Chronic inflammation is a huge problem in our society that contributes to many non-infectious diseases including heart disease, cancer, Alzheimer's, autoimmune disease, and more, according to the National Center for Biotechnology Information.

Diet and lifestyle play a huge part in chronic inflammation but when folks are already eating a healthy, nutrient-dense diet and optimizing their lifestyle (getting enough sleep and exercise for example), CBD oil can help. Research also shows that CBD oil can reduce chronic inflammation that leads to disease.

Other Remedies to Consider: Research agrees that it is important to address gut health to manage inflammation. Removing refined sugar from the diet has also been shown to reduce inflammation in as little as a week.

6. Reduces Oxidative Stress

Oxidative stress is responsible for many ailments today. Oxidative stress is when the body has too many free radicals and can't keep up with neutralizing them (with antioxidants). This is more of a problem now than in the past because our environment is so much more toxic than it once was. A 2010 study shows that CBD oil acts as an antioxidant and another study found CBD has neuroprotective qualities. So CBD can reduce neurological damage caused by free radicals.

7. Help for Schizophrenia

Schizophrenia is a complicated and serious disease that is typically managed through therapy and pharmaceutical drugs (that carry hefty side effects). Anecdotally, many folks have found that CBD oil has helped reduce hallucinations. Research is beginning to catch up too. A March 2015 review of available research found that CBD was a safe, effective, and well tolerated treatment for psychosis. But more research is needed to bring CBD into clinical practice.

It should be mentioned that THC, the psychoactive compound in marijuana, may actually increase psychosis for those at risk. CBD oil, on the other hand, only helps reduce psychosis and may even counteract psychosis brought on by marijuana use.

8. Promotes Healthy Weight

Cannabidiol can help maintain healthy blood sugar, stimulates genes and proteins that helps break down fat, and increase mitochondria that helps burn calories.

CBD also encourages the body to convert white fat to brown fat. White fat is the kind of fat we typically think of when we think about body fat. Brown fat is fat that is in small deposits that behaves differently than white fat. Brown fat is said to improve health by enhancing the bodies ability to burn white fat, create heat, and even regulate blood sugar.

9. Improves Heart Health

Heart disease is a growing problem today. In fact, it's the leading cause of death in the U.S. A healthy diet and lifestyle is a top priority for heart health, but CBD oil can also help. According to research cannabidiol reduces artery blockage, reduces stress induced cardiovascular response, and can reduce blood pressure. It may also reduce cholesterol.

As mentioned earlier, CBD oil is helpful in preventing oxidative stress and inflammation. Both of these are often precursors to heart disease.

10. Improves Skin Conditions

CBD oil can be used topically to treat skin conditions. Studies show CBD oil has a high potential for treating skin conditions like eczema by encouraging abnormal cell death. It can also help regulate the skin's oil production, reducing acne. CBD also contains many nutrients like vitamin E that help improve and protect the skin.

Other Remedies to Consider: Diet is vitally important for skin health. Many people find that removing foods like sugar, dairy or grains (if sensitive) improves skin. I also personally use a skin probiotic spray that has made a huge difference for my acne prone skin.

11. Fights Cancer

CBD oil's role in cancer treatment still needs more research, but what is available is looking promising. According to the American Cancer Society, CBD oil can slow growth and spread of some kinds of cancer (in animals). Because it fights oxidative stress and inflammation (and both are linked to cancer) it makes sense that CBD oil could help fight cancer cells.

This is a common question and misconception. As mentioned above, while they come from the same plant, they are different strains and CBD is harvested from the plants that contain no THC (or negligible levels). CBD is completely legal and is not considered a drug. Because of the often confused history of these plants, many manufacturers use "hemp oil" instead of the more controversial "CBD oil" in their marketing. CBD levels can vary drastically based on manufacturing, so it is important to find a high quality manufacturer with verified levels.

From a sustainability standpoint, it is a shame that hemp has gotten so much negative press because it comes from a similar strain of plant. Aside from the CBD benefits, hemp is one of the strongest, longest, and most durable natural fibers and it can be grown without any type of pesticides or herbicides! It also:

Makes up to four times as much fiber per acre as pine trees

Can be recycled many more times than pine-based pulp products

Is easy to grow without chemicals and is actually good for the soil

Produces a seed and seed oil rich in protein, essential fatty acids and amino acids

CBD oil is most often used internally (through ingestion). Because CBD oil is a relatively new supplement, exact dosing isn't well established. While more long-term studies are needed, there is no established CBD "overdose" and there are very few if any side effects at any dosage.

When trying to find the right dosage, consider these things:

Start by purchasing a high quality oil from a reputable company. A higher quality oil will be more bioavailable, so a lower dose can be enough.

Begin with the recommended dosage on the bottle (especially if using preventatively).

Some notice a change immediately, while others don't notice any improvement for several weeks. If after several weeks there is still no change, increase the dosage.

As with most herbal supplements, a small dosage 3-4 times a day is usually more therapeutic than one large dose.

Though CBD oil on its own is very safe, it may interact with medications, particularly opioids. Speak with your doctor if you're concerned about interactions or are unsure about using hemp oil for your conditions. I know it's tough to find a primary care doctor who understands alternative practices, but there are options like this service that pair you with a doctor who fits your lifestyle.

CBD Oil for Pets

Sidenote for our furrier friends: All mammals have an endocannabinoid system, CBD oil can have some of the same benefits for pets as it does for humans.

For cats and dogs in particular, CBD oil may help with:

excessive barking or crying

pets getting along with other pets

pain

relaxing pets before a trip to the vet

lack of appetite

separation anxiety

There may be some trial and error in finding the right dosage for pets. Start with a low dose of 1 milligrams per 10 pounds of body weight and go up to 5 milligrams per 10 pounds of body weight if needed. A higher dose may be necessary for some ailments. A low dose 3-4 times a day is usually more therapeutic than one large dose.

CBD: What I've Tried (& What I Will)

There are lots of benefits to using CBD oil as a supplement. A healthy diet and lifestyle should always be the first step to improved health, but CBD oil can help build on that foundation.

CBD Hemp Oil – A Natural Way to Perfect Health

Does CBD Really Work For Anxiety?

Anxiety affects almost all of us in small ways. Before giving a speech or doing something new, we might feel unsure, unprepared or nervous. Some of those feelings may well manifest in physical symptoms like shortness of breath, clammy hands or headaches.

However, to people who have been diagnosed with an anxiety disorder or who experience panic attacks, anxiety is so much more than simply feeling overwhelmed. It can be totally debilitating.

Typical treatments for anxiety usually center around either therapy, medication or both. This includes talk therapy or cognitive behavioral therapy, and medications like benzodiazepines, antidepressants, beta blockers and SNRIs (serotonin and norepinephrine reuptake inhibitors). But non-pharmaceutical solutions are also becoming more popular, especially as new research on them emerges. Case in point: CBD products.

CBD, or cannabidiol, comes from the cannabis plant. This plant produces over 400 different chemicals, one of which is CBD. CBD products on their own contain little to no THC, the psychoactive component found in the plant that makes users feel high or stoned. This, however, doesn't make the product totally free to use without legal repercussions anywhere you want: CBD may still be classified as an illegal substance in some states, although the law is often murky and up for interpretation.

CBD is available in oils, or it can be added to creams, ointments and beauty products. It can also be used in a vape pen or even consumed through food like CBD gummies. Joel Greengrass, CEO of Theramu, a company that creates non-THC CBD oil and observed a huge increase in interest popularity of CBD for skin and wellness complaints, as well as for the treatment of a range of anxiety conditions.

"Overall awareness of CBD and the variety of ailments and symptoms that it can relieve is increasing daily as is the desire to move away from harsh prescription pharmaceuticals."

Is CBD Hemp Oil the Answer to Perfect Health?

Because of all of the great stories out there that show how CBD Hemp oil is helping lots and lots of people with hard health problems we can honestly say that YES. CBD Hemp Oil is indeed one of the answers to perfect health.

Interesting Facts about the Hemp Plant

Hemp is one of the oldest plants known to man. It dates from 8.000 BC and it commonly refers to the industrial varieties of Cannabis plant and its products: fiber, oil and seed.

Apart from its medicinal use, hemp has an industrial one as well. Throughout history, it is known to be contained in:

- foods
- hemp oil
- CBD hemp oil
- wax
- resin
- rope
- cloth
- pulp
- paper
- fuel
- and more

Hemp plant is easy to grow and it actually improves the soil in which it grows. It grows very quickly and it can grow up to five meters. It has very versatile fiber because of the high amount of cellulose. It basically makes everything stronger and better, which is why it has so many industrial applications.

How is CBD Hemp Oil made?

CBD oil can be extracted in three ways:

Super or Sub-critical CO_2 method

This is extracting oil in high pressure and low temperature. CO2 is pushed through the plant and the result is CBD in its purest form. It is considered as the best and safest method, the extracted CBD-rich hemp oil has clean taste because the green chlorophyll is removed during the extraction. This method is more expensive than the alternatives and requires expensive equipment.

Solvent extraction method

CBD hemp oil is extracted by so called Rectified spirit (also known as neutral spirit, rectified alcohol, or ethyl alcohol of agricultural origin). With this method it's super important to use only highly concentrated ethanol which has been purified by means of repeated distillation.

Neutral spirits can be produced from grain, grapes, sugar beets, sugarcane, or other fermented plant material.

Oil method or Carrier Oil Extraction

A popular method based on extraction by a carrier oil, usually olive oil. It is save and there is no unwanted, harmful residue in the extracted oil. There's just one downside to this method: carrier oils have a short shelf life. Therefore, CBD hemp oil made in this way should be stored in smaller amounts and ingested orally.

As soon as you realize that you are responsible for your own well-being and you deserve a good, healthy life, you should definitely try CBD Hemp Oil. You'll discover that it can do miracles for you. There are so many ways in which it has already proved to be effective and many more are yet to be proven.

Here are some of the effects of CBD hemp oil explained in more detail:

Anxiety and stress

Endocannabinoids (ECS) are chemical compounds that play a key role in memory, mood, brain reward systems, drug addiction, and energy balance. They are activated by the same receptors as CBD. Research shows the benefits of the ECS system in fighting depression, anxiety, increasing appetite, and creating feelings of well-being. CBD naturally acts on the ECS system's signals to increase receptor function and flow.

Anti-Inflammatory and pain-relief effects

The extent to which this oil can help with inflammation, starting from joint pain to irritable bowel syndrome to diabetic retinopathy, are absolutely astonishing! CBD hemp oil is much more powerful than many of the commonly recommend natural remedies for inflammation.

Reduction of seizures

Cannabis was first used to treat epilepsy back in 1800 B.C.E. In 2014 the FDA moved forward with allowing the drug Epidiolex, a 99% oil-based extract of CBD for fighting childhood epilepsy. Results showed that there was a 54% decrease in seizures in 137 people who were on Epidiolex for 12 weeks. Those tested had no success with any prior treatment, and of the 25 patients who had Dravet syndrome, there was a 63% decrease in seizures over the course of three months.

Increases appetite

With patients who undergo chemotherapy, one of the biggest problems they face is loss of appetite. CBD hemp oil can help them regain their appetite. Medication, illnesses, and mental reaction to illnesses causes loss of appetite. Throughout history, CBD has shown itself to encourage appetite.Proper nourishment means a lot for people who fight with difficult diseases and conditions.

Anti-Psychotic Effects

Research suggests that CBD is able to prevent psychotic episodes that are usually associated with THC. Research shows that CBD may be able to provide therapeutic relief in various forms of psychosis, with schizophrenia being the most prominent. CBD has reportedly been shown to treat schizophrenia with little side effects. The other drugs used for treating this disease have many side-effects.

Anti-Cancer Properties

Anti-Cancer study from 2013 showed that CBD was able to trigger necessary apoptosis and autophagy in cancer cells. Scientists from the study were able to attack breast cancer cells and inhibit further cancer cell growth. There have also been reports of parents who provide CBD to their children in order to achieve cancer remission.

Anti-Bacterial

CBD hemp oil can also provide antibacterial protection for the body. CBD has been used as a treatment for tuberculosis and other diseases since 1950. It is also able to fight forms of staphylococci and streptococci infections which many modern antibiotics are unable to. With the overuse of antibiotics today, bacteria begin to evolve and become very reisstant to prescribed antibiotics – CBD's antibacterial properties can come in handy.

Neurodegenerative Disorders

These disorders can be caused by inflammation of the brain, and as CBD can reduce inflammation, it can reportedly help with the following disoireds: Alzheimer's disease, Huntington's disease, and MS all lead to degeneration of the brain. However, use of CBD can increase activity in the ECS system and lower the risk of common neurological diseases.

It also works for:

Balancing Hormones

Balancing Weight

Antibiotic-resistant infections

Rheumatoid arthritis

Psoriasis

PTSD (Post Traumatic Stress Disorder)

Vascular and muscle relaxing

Diabetes

Alcoholism

Spasms

Dosage – How much CBD Hemp Oil Should You Take?

Considering all the different ways in which CBD hemp oil works, it is very hard to set one standard dosage for every disease and every person. You need to have all the criteria in mind.

Dosage depends on:

Kind of disease or condition

Severity of the disease or the condition

Progression of the disease of the disease or the condition

Body weight

Age

It also matters that CBD hemp oil comes in various forms and concentrations, including:

Liquid oil

Oil in the form of a thick paste (aka CBD Extract)

- Tincture
- Oil in capsules
- Drops or sprays
- Salves for topical use
- CBD vapor
- CBD in Chocolates, candies, gums

Cbd-hemp-oil-cannabidiol

All things considered, the best way to go is start small and then increase the dosage as you go on.

The duration of the treatment depends on the disease.

A very important fact: there aren't ANY known side-effects from the usage of CBD hemp oil.

The most effective way to go is find out more about the CBD hemp oil from your provider/seller and ask for more detailed instructions on the dosage.

In our store we sell CBD Hemp oil that we actually make from the ground up. We don't like to resell something that we have no idea how it was made. So we make our own products.

Our CBD oil drops are all the same for the ease of use – they contain 400mg of CBD in every 10ml. So the bigger the bottle the more CBD is mixed in. We mix it with Hemp Seed oil.

Recommended dosage for an adult person of average height and weight male or female:

- for light issues like high blood pressure: 3 drops in the morning and 5 drops before sleep for issues like diabetes, asthma, etc: 5 drops in the morning, 5 drops at lunch and 10 drops before sleep

for hard issues like cancer: 10 drops in the morning, 10 drops at lunch and 20 drops before sleep

Now this is just to give you some idea.

To get a precise recommendation please email us and we will be more then happy to help!

CBD Hemp Oil – Give it a chance, give yourself a chance

After everything you've learned about this amazing, life-changing CBD hemp oil, I believe you'll give it a try.

If you suffer from an aggressive disease which consumes all your life energy, the oil will help you regain control of your own destiny.

CBD Oil for Anxiety: Treating Anxiety Disorders Safely

In America alone, 40 million people suffer annually from anxiety disorders, and this number continues to grow. Anxiety is more than just sweaty palms and stress dreams before a big test or interview. It's a crippling mental disorder that can make even simple, daily tasks seem huge and overwhelming.

Anxiety doesn't just affect the brain — it has profound and long-lasting effects on the body as well. Common side effects of anxiety include:

Difficulty sleeping

Numbness or tingling, usually in the hands

Decreased blood flow

- Shortness of breath
- Muscle tension
- Nausea
- Gastrointestinal inflammation and discomfort
- Dizziness
- Headaches
- Flushed skin

Big Pharma's Anxiety Solutions

When people are diagnosed with an anxiety or stress disorder, the first thing that most medical practitioners do is turn to pharmaceutical solutions. Medications such as Prozac, Xanax, and Valium are the most common prescriptions, but these carry a host of harmful side effects and may quickly become addictive.

CBD oil has been shown to be a promising alternative therapy, with the same properties as antidepressants and anxiolytics, but without the numerous risks. Studies show that anxiety can be significantly reduced by CBD. In fact, CBD oil works faster than most anti-anxiety medications. For those who struggle with situational anxiety and panic attacks, this quick response-time can be life-changing.

How Does CBD Oil Reduce Anxiety?

CBD oil affects your body through your endocannabinoid system, which is made up of cannabinoid receptors. These little protein receptors are specifically designed to respond to cannabinoids, whether those your own body produces or those you obtain from plants. You have these receptors all over your body, including your skin and even in your intestines!

Your endocannabinoid system is involved in controlling inflammation, pain, sleep, immune function, mood, brain function (such as memory), hunger, and even reproduction.

CBD oil for anxiety control improves symptoms of:

Generalized anxiety

Panic disorders

Social fears and phobias

PTSD

Obsessive Compulsive Disorder (OCD)

Mild depression

While more research needs to be done to fully understand how CBD oil for anxiety is effective, research has shown that cannabinoids influence serotonin receptors, such as 5-HT1A. When more serotonin is available in the brain, more neurons are activated. When more neurons are activated, mood is improved and anxiety is reduced.

But CBD oil does more than just activate neurons — it also encourages new neurons to be created, called neurogenesis. CBD has been shown to encourage neurogenesis in the hippocampus, the part of your brain that regulates emotions and forms memories.

Brain scans have shown that those who suffer from anxiety disorders often have a smaller hippocampus than others who do not struggle with anxiety. When new neurons are created in the hippocampus, anxiety and depression symptoms improve.

Things You Should Know About Using CBD Oil for Anxiety and Depression

It's important to understand two things about using CBD oil for anxiety.

First, CBD oil is NOT the same as THC, which is the component in cannabis responsible for the 'high.' CBD oil is non-psychoactive. It will not make you high. CBD oil contains trace amounts of THC — .3% to be exact — but this is not even remotely close enough to produce a high.

Secondly, CBD oil is not a sedation drug. This means that you can use CBD oil without worrying that it will affect your mental state. Other types of antidepressants can suppress emotions, giving a feeling of emotional 'flatness. They can also cause a feeling of 'fuzziness,' or a dream-like state. CBD oil does not affect the body in these ways.

A large dose of CBD oil can make you feel sleepy, but this is easily avoided by taking lower doses.

It's said that humans are born with only two fears — the fear of falling, and the fear of loud noises. All the rest are fears that develop as we age. Whether your anxiety is from a chemical imbalance, a traumatic event, or another source, CBD oil may be the natural, safe solution to help you regain control of your emotional life.

CBD Oil for Anxiety: Social Fears and Phobias

Have a high-stress job with an important pitch or presentation coming up? The fear of public speaking or intimidating social interactions is one of the most common forms of anxiety. For some, social anxiety simply makes parties, work gatherings, or a daily job uncomfortable and exhausting. For others with social anxiety, it is a crippling fear that keeps them locked indoors and in isolation.

For the rest of us? We're probably dealing with situational anxiety, such as that before a big business meeting, an interview, a first date, or a public speaking engagement.

CBD oil can help with all of this. CBD oil taken before a stressful social situation significantly reduced the following:

Anxiety

- Elevated heart rate
- Trembling
- Shaking knees
- Sweating
- Dry mouth
- Shaking voice
- Inability to form thoughts (aka cognitive impairment)
- Lack of alertness

CBD Oil for Panic Attacks

CBD oil works by balancing our autonomic nervous system — or, in other words, it chills us out when we're on the brink of a nervous breakdown. Think of it as a nervous system reset. CBD oil produces a chemical calming of the sympathetic branch of your nervous system.

To use preventatively, administer CBD oil before walking into a potentially nerve-wracking situation. If your trauma has caught you unawares, administer CBD oil in the midst of a panic attack to help your body naturally (and quickly) calm down.

At some point, we all need a mood booster. For some, depression is an area we struggle with regularly.

CBD oil can help control the sympathetic branch of your nervous system, helping those with nervous disorders better manage mood. CBD oil can help you regulate your emotional responses by reducing anxiety and hysteria. When anxiety goes down, mood goes up.

CBD Oil for Anxiety Induced Insomnia

Who hasn't been through a period in their lives in which the overwhelming stress and worry of daily life caused an inability to sleep?

This lack of sleep causes a vicious cycle of anxiety and exhaustion, as one triggers or worsens the other.

CBD oil can help to stop this vicious cycle in its tracks by tackling both problems with one safe solution. As CBD oil reduces anxiety throughout the day, the mind and body are able to relax and fall asleep. But CBD oil is also used to help treat insomnia — which means more sleep, and less stress.

CBD Oil for Post Traumatic Stress Disorder (PTSD)

The British Pharmacological Society claims CBD oil can reduce learned fear responses. This is a huge opportunity for those who suffer from PTSD. Studies showed that CBD was able to:

Reduce fear expression

Smooth disrupted memory

Aid in enhancing memory

Diminish fears and the panic attacks associated with PTSD

In a lab protocol designed to mimic PTSD, CBD oil improved patients abilities to forget and release traumatic memories. This would allow individuals to move on from past traumatic events, giving them the freedom to rebuild their lives.

CBD Oil Anxiety Relief FAQ's

The following are just a few of the questions from our customers lately. If you've got a question you don't see an answer to here, call either of our store locations.

Almost nil! This is one of the best benefits of CBD oil for anxiety relief! CBD oil causes no serious side effects. There are a few minor discomforts you may experience, however.

Dry mouth

- Mild nausea

- Drowsiness (lessen dose or change CBD oil blend)

Please keep in mind that CBD oil may interfere with other prescription medications, so be sure to consult your physician before taking CBD oil.

Is using CBD oil for anxiety addictive?

Nope! CBD oil is a non-addictive substance.

Can CBD oil get you high?

No. CBD oil does not contain tetrahydrocannabinol (THC) which is the psychoactive component responsible for producing a 'high'. True CBD oil cannot get you high.

There are a few great products out there. At Apple Wellness, our favorite brands are Charlotte's Web and CBD Plus. Whatever brand you choose, make sure that you find a product made from highest-grade CBD oil. Do your research, because CBD oil knockoffs are out there. They won't do you any good and may do you harm.

Should I try using CBD oil for anxiety or depression?

If you suffer from anxiety or depression, we strongly recommend investigating CBD oil as a treatment option. This is safe, natural, and non-addictive. The best thing to do is to stop by one of our stores or give us a call. We can talk through your needs to find the best CBD oil for anxiety relief.

How do I determine the correct CBD oil dosage for anxiety?

Start with the smallest recommended dose on your CBD oil product, and gradually increase it until you experience the desired effect. Finding the best CBD oil dosage for anxiety can take several days to a couple of weeks. All of our bodies and situations are different, and finding the best balance may take time. For quickest results, talk to one of our Wellness Consultants.

Benefits of CBD Oil (Cannabidiol) & Why It's Not What You Think.

The medical use of marijuana has brought some attention to the subject of using cannabis-derived products for health, but it's important to understand how CBD oil differs. We'll get into this more in a bit, but the key difference lies in the parts of the plant being used to make the product. For example, CBD oil is also different from hemp seed oil, since it is extracted not from the seed but from the flowers, leaves, and stalks of hemp.

Surprisingly, research shows that CBD products are actually helpful at reducing many ailments. Such diverse ailments that they seem to be unrelated, in fact… but they are not. Emerging research shows that each of these ailments may be related to dysregulation of the endocannabinoid system, or ECS for short.

Haven't heard of it? You're not alone! It's not as familiar to us as the cardiovascular or immune system, but is a critical component of the human body.

Understanding the Endocannabinoid System

The endocannabinoid system is possibly one of the most fascinating systems in the body. It was discovered through researching the effects of cannabis on the body. In fact, this amazing system that regulates the body's internal balance got its name from the cannabis plant that made its discovery possible.

The endocannabinoid system is made up of endocannabinoids and their receptors. These are found everywhere in the body from the brain and other organs to glands and immune cells. The endocannabinoid system works differently in different parts of the body but the end goal is homeostasis (internal balance).

Ever heard of a "runner's high"? Research reported in the Scientific American found endocannabinoids are largely responsible for this natural "hit" of euphoria that increases feelings of well-being and decreases the perception of pain.

Cannabidiol (CBD oil) is another way to affect this powerful body system ... but am I really saying "getting high" is a good thing?

It turns out there's a very important distinction still to be made ...

Does CBD Oil Create a High?

The short answer is: No. (Though oils with THC can also contain CBD).

There are two different types of CBD oil products — hemp-based CBD oil (the one I'm talking about in this book) and marijuana-based CBD (which is what someone would buy at the dispensary). Both contain CBD, and they're both derived from the cannabis plant, but hemp and medical marijuana are are different varieties of the plant.

Marijuana-based CBD is generally going to have more THC and other cannabinoids. CBD oil does not contain THC (the compound that causes a "high" feeling). This is an important distinction that many people don't understand.

The variety that is typically (and legally) used to make CBD oil is hemp. How is hemp oil different? A plant can only be legally considered hemp if it contains .3% per dry unit (or less) of the compound THC.

In a nutshell, CBD oil or hemp oil contains the benefits of the cannabis plant without the potential drawbacks of psychoactive compounds typically found from inhalation or other methods of consumption.

How Can You Treat Anxiety with Cannabis Oil?

Everyone gets anxious from time to time. It is a normal emotion.

But anxiety disorders are different. They are a group of mental illnesses, and the difficulty they cause can cause disruptions to a person's day-to-day life.

People who have an anxiety disorder have fears and worries that are overwhelming, constant, and even disabling.

Types of Anxiety Disorders

Anxiety disorder is a general term that includes a number of different conditions including the following:

Social Anxiety Disorder

This is also known as a social phobia where individuals feel self-consciousness and overwhelming worry about normal, everyday social situations. They focus on others judging them or being ridiculed or embarrassed.

Panic Disorder

Individuals feel terror that strikes at random. During a panic attack, they may have chest pain, sweat, and feel palpitations (which are irregular or unusually strong heartbeats). They may also feel like they are choking or experiencing a heart attack.

Phobias

Individuals feel an intense fear of a specific situation or object, such as spiders or heights. The fear goes above what is appropriate and may even cause individuals to avoid ordinary situations.

Generalized Anxiety Disorder

Individuals feel unrealistic, excessive tension and worry with little or no reason to explain why.

Researchers still do not know exactly what brings on anxiety disorders. They arise from a combination of things including environmental stress, changes in the brain, and even genetics.

Symptoms of Anxiety Disorders

General symptoms of anxiety disorders include the following:

- Sleep problems
- Fear, panic, and uneasiness
- Shortness of breath
- Tense muscles
- Dry mouth
- Dizziness
- Not being able to stay still or calm
- Heart palpitations
- Cold, numb, sweaty or tingling hands or feet

But, how can you treat anxiety?

CBD for Anxiety

Early research shows encouraging signs that cannabis may relieve anxiety. CBD is a type of cannabinoid, which is a natural chemical compound found in cannabis plants.

Cannabis oil is said to work with a brain receptor known as CB1. These receptors are tiny proteins attached to a person's cells. They help the cells respond to chemical signals from different stimuli.

Although not completely understood how CBD affects the CB1 receptor, it is thought that it alters serotonin signals. It is the serotonin that plays a role in your mental health, and not having enough of it can cause anxiety for many people.

The conventional treatment of low serotonin levels is selective serotonin reuptake inhibitors, such as Prozac or Zoloft. But for many people, cannabis oil is a natural, alternative way to manage anxiety.

How Much CBD Oil Should I Take for Anxiety?

Anxiety is an unpleasant issue that many people struggle with. While occasional anxiety is completely normal, it's when worrying thoughts begin to spiral out of control that anxiety poses real problems. At its most severe, anxiety can have profound negative effects on your life. It can even prevent you from taking part in daily activities you may take for granted.

But just because you have anxiety, it doesn't need to impact your life ☐uite so much. Many people are finding relief with an alternative natural remedy called CBD oil, as it helps to manage anxious feelings and thoughts.

Anxiety is a form of mental illness that includes panic disorder, obsessive-compulsive disorder (OCD), general anxiety disorder, and social anxiety disorder. It affects around 40 million adults in the U.S., or 18.1% of the population every year. If you are currently suffering from anxiety, then take strength in the fact that you are not alone.

The condition is characterized by feelings of dread or worry, often over some future event. It is different from fear, which is a response to a real or perceived threat. Anxiety can make you uneasy, overly worried, and restless. It is also commonly accompanied by tension in the muscles and problems concentrating.

But not all anxiety is bad. In fact, anxiety is a natural adaptation that helps humans to avoid danger. It is one of the main reasons that our species has survived and thrived for so long. It is when these feelings are not managed effectively that it can become a problem.

Symptoms of anxiety

Recognizing that you have anxiety is the first step in getting it under control. In order to do that, take a look at these common symptoms of anxiety and see if they commonly affect you.

Excessive worry

Rumination (constantly going over negative thoughts in your head)

Feelings of dread or uneasiness

Muscular tension

Fatigue

Problems concentrating

Poor sleep

Somatic complaints (like butterflies in stomach or indigestion)

These factors have led to CBD oil becoming a hugely popular alternative treatment for a wide range of conditions, including anxiety.

How can CBD oil reduce anxiety?

There has been a fair amount of research into CBD and its effects on anxiety. While most of the studies are conducted on animal subjects, CBD does show great promise in this area. However, much more research needs to be done, especially in a clinical setting.

What the research has found is that CBD oil may work to relieve anxiety by acting upon serotonin pathways in the brain. Serotonin is a chemical that transmits messages between nerve cells in the brain. It contributes to your overall mood and wellbeing.

By acting as a 5-HT1 receptor agonist, CBD may boost signalling through serotonin receptors and enhance the production of serotonin. This animal study seems to support that theory. The Spanish researchers even noted that CBD may affect serotonin faster than traditional antidepressant medication (SSRIs) that are commonly prescribed for anxiety.

Research into CBD and anxiety

Over recent years, CBD has garnered a lot of interest among patients, doctors. and scientists. And with good reason. A number of scientific studies have shown CBD to have powerful anti-anxiety properties. It is also proven to be incredibly safe and well-tolerated, even at high doses.

As a result, many people are doing away with their traditional anxiety medication and the side-effects that come with it and turning to CBD oil to help relieve the symptoms of their anxiety.

Anxiety symptoms in people with social anxiety disorder. This research also found that cannabidiol altered the way participants responded to anxiety, which may be due to changes in blood flow in regions of the brain associated with feelings of anxiety.

Further research has also concluded that cannabidiol is effective in treating anxiety – this may be why CBD oil is popular with anxiety sufferers. A 2014 study revealed that CBD oil possessed anti-anxiety and anti-depressant effects (in an animal model).

Cannabidiol could diminish post-traumatic stress disorder symptoms and anxiety provoked sleep disorder in a child patient with a background of trauma. The researchers discovered that cannabidiol helped to reduce anxiety in the child, as well as helping to improve sleep.

CBD Oil Vs antidepressants

The most commonly prescribed antidepressants for anxiety are known as SSRIs. Like CBD, SSRIs also act on serotonin receptors in the brain to reduce the symptoms of anxiety. The main downside with these medications, however, is the side effects that they produce.

These side effects can include drowsiness, insomnia, and sexual problems. This means SSRIs are not advisable to take on a long-term basis. They also don't work for everyone. Some studies suggest that antidepressants such as SSRIs work only work on about half of people who take them.

Cannabis, on the other hand, has been used medically in the west for over 100 years, and for more than 4,000 years in the east. Most remarkably, in all this time, not one death has been attributed to cannabis.

Unlike regular cannabis, which is now illegal in much of the world, CBD oil is completely legal and available for sale. This is because CBD oil doesn't produce any harmful effects, making it safe to use with minimal side effects.

CBD oil is currently being used by many anxiety sufferers as it has been shown to have potent anti-anxiety and antidepressant qualities. And being perfectly legal to use and non-intoxicating, CBD oil is suitable for everyone. Unlike many prescription medications, using CBD oil for anxiety doesn't result in side effects like low libido or feeling overly sedated.

How Much CBD For Anxiety?

A ꙮuestion that is often asked by new users is how much CBD oil should you take for anxiety. The answer is that it varies. This is because CBD acts very differently in each individual. Therefore, it's highly important to consider how much CBD to take before you start using it.

As we all have a uniꙮue physiology, finding the correct amount of CBD oil will be personal to you. Your height and weight can also play a part in selecting the correct dosage. If you have a medical condition, its best to consult your doctor before taking CBD oil.

So, how much CBD is best for anxiety? Ideally, starting with a low dose and building up is the way forward for most new users. As there are no official guidelines set in stone yet, time and patience are the keys to determining the most effective dose for you. Here are some points to keep in mind.

Before you start taking CBD for anxiety, consider your weight and how severe your condition is.

You could start with just one drop of CBD oil on your first day of use. This low dose gives your body time to adapt to the CBD and ensures you're not going to take too much.

Slowly increase your dosage. You may wish to increase your dose to 2 drops per day for a few weeks to see if you notice any visible reduction in your anxiety symptoms. It will take time for CBD to affect you, so changes can take a while to notice. Before increasing your dose, stick with the same amount of CBD for at least a few days.

Separate your dosage into smaller doses throughout the day. This may enhance the absorption rate and efficacy of the CBD oil.

Speak to your doctor before you take CBD oil for anxiety, especially if you are already on medication. Using a CBD tincture may increase the potency of other drugs. If you're taking prescription medication and want to reduce or stop your drug, speak to a qualified healthcare worker first.

From research and information published online from users of CBD oil, doses between 40mg and 600mg seem most effective. A study on social anxiety and CBD oil found that a dose of 600mg was effective in reducing anxiety. However, other studies have found that lower doses are also effective in diminishing the symptoms of anxiety.

While it is difficult to suggest a specific dose of CBD, using the following chart can help to determine a suitable starting dose.

Side effects of CBD

It's important to consider the side effects of any supplement to your daily diet. CBD oil may hinder hepatic drug metabolism and the activity of some enzymes in the liver. Some users may also find they have a dry mouth after usage.

However, the majority of research studies on CBD have demonstrated little or no side effects. This review reveals that standard use is safe for humans.

You can purchase various kinds of CBD oils, but choosing a high-quality product from a trustworthy brand will ensure you the best chance of positive effects.

A high-quality product like our very own Good Vibes 250+ CBD oil enriched with vitamins and omega fatty acids is a good choice. Made from organically grown hemp, this expertly developed supplement will help you to discover why CBD oil is so popular with many of our customers.

Final thoughts on CBD oil and anxiety

Anxiety is a common mental health issue that many people suffer from. Although it is a natural adaptation that allows us to anticipate danger, anxiety can cause untold amounts of distress when not kept under control.

It's also a very complex condition. The causes of anxiety are often simplified, but in truth can be wide-ranging. This means that treating anxiety is often not as simple as prescribing a pill. A more holistic approach is best. And CBD oil can play a big help in restoring you, your mind, and your body back to full health.

CBD has been shown in numerous scientific studies to reduce anxiety and depression. Many people are finding relief in this extremely safe, non-intoxicating supplement. A lot of them are even finding it an effective replacement for traditional medication such as antidepressants and SSRIs.

However, there is still much research to be done on the subject. While the results of studies that have been done are promising, a complete understanding of how CBD works to reduce anxiety is needed.

Until then, it's worth seeing if CBD oil can help you. Try our Good Vibes 250+ CBD oil today and join the ever-growing trend of regular people that are using CBD oil to combat their anxiety.

Here's what you need to know about six potential medical uses of CBD and where the research stands:

1. Anxiety relief

CBD may be able to help you manage anxiety. Researchers think it may change the way your brain's receptors respond to serotonin, a chemical linked to mental health. Receptors are tiny proteins attached to your cells that receive chemical messages and help your cells respond to different stimuli.

One study found that a 600mg dose of CBD helped people with social anxiety give a speech. Other early studies done with animals have shown that CBD may help relieve anxiety by:

Reducing stress

Decreasing physiological effects of anxiety, such as an increased heart rate

Improving symptoms of post-traumatic stress disorder (PTSD)

Inducing sleep in cases of insomnia

2. Anti-seizure

CBD has been in the news before, as a possible treatment for epilepsy. Research is still in its early days. Researchers are testing how much CBD is able to reduce the number of seizures in people with epilepsy, as well as how safe it is. The American Epilepsy Society states that cannabidiol research offers hope for seizure disorders, and that research is currently being conducted to better understand safe use.

3. Neuroprotective

Researchers are looking at a receptor located in the brain to learn about the ways that CBD could help people with neurodegenerative disorders, which are diseases that cause the brain and nerves to deteriorate over time. This receptor is known as CB1.

Researchers are studying the use of CBD oil for treating:

Alzheimer's disease

multiple sclerosis (MS)

Parkinson's disease

stroke

CBD oil may also reduce the inflammation that can make neurodegenerative symptoms worse. More research is needed to fully understand the effects of CBD oil for neurodegenerative diseases.

4. Pain relief

The effects of CBD oil on your brain's receptors may also help you manage pain. Studies have shown that cannabis can offer some benefits when taken after chemotherapy treatments. Other pre-clinical studies sponsored by the National Institutes of Health are also looking at the role of cannabis in relieving symptoms caused by:

arthritis

chronic pain

- MS pain
- muscle pain
- spinal cord injuries

Nabiximols (Sativex), a multiple sclerosis drug made from a combination of TCH and CBD, is approved in the United Kingdom and Canada to treat MS pain. However, researchers think the CBD in the drug may be contributing more with its anti-inflammatory properties than by acting against the pain. Clinical trials of CBD are necessary to determine whether or not it should be used for pain management.

5. Anti-acne

The effects of CBD on receptors in the immune system may help reduce overall inflammation in the body. In turn, CBD oil may offer benefits for acne management. A human study published in the Journal of Clinical Investigation found that the oil prevented activity in sebaceous glands. These glands are responsible for producing sebum, a natural oily substance that hydrates the skin. Too much sebum, however, can lead to acne.

Before you consider CBD oil for acne treatment, it's worth discussing with your dermatologist. More human studies are needed to evaluate the potential benefits of CBD for acne.

5. Cancer treatment

Some studies have investigated the role of CBD in preventing cancer cell growth, but research is still in its early stages. The National Cancer Institute (NCI) says that CBD may help alleviate cancer symptoms and cancer treatment side effects. However, the NCI doesn't fully endorse any form of cannabis as a cancer treatment. The action of CBD that's promising for cancer treatment is its ability to moderate inflammation and change how cell reproduce. CBD has the effect of reducing the ability of some types of tumor cells to reproduce.

Cannabidiol effective works for treating anxiety

CBD experts dealing in effective pain relief through the use of legal hemp derived cannabidiol products.

While we don't normally think of anxiety as desirable, it's actually a critical adaptive response that can help us cope with threats to our (or a loved one's) safety and welfare. These responses help us recognize and avert potential threats; they can also help motivate us to take action to better our situation (work harder, pay bills, improve relationships, etc.). However, when we don't manage these natural responses effectively, they can become maladaptive and impact our work and relationships. This can lead to clinically diagnosable anxiety-related disorders. We've all heard the saying, "stress kills." It's true!

Anxiety-related disorders affect a huge segment of our population—40 million adults (18%) in the United States age 18 and older. In response, Big Pharma has developed numerous drugs to treat anxiety-related disorders, from selective serotonin reuptake inhibitors (SSRIs) like Prozac and Zoloft to tranquilizers (the most popular class being benzodiazepines such as Valium and Xanax).

While these drugs can be effective for many patients, some don't respond favorably. Certain patients don't see much improvement, or they can't tolerate the side effects. Moreover, tranquilizers like Valium and Xanax can be highly addictive. Clearly, alternative treatments are warranted. Could cannabidiol (CBD), the most prominent non-intoxicating constituent in cannabis, provide a viable alternative for currently available anxiety medications? Quite possibly!

In recent years, CBD has generated a tremendous amount of interest among consumers, clinicians, and scientists. Why? Not only does evidence suggest CBD counteracts many of THC's adverse effects, but numerous animal studies and accumulating evidence from human experimental, clinical, and epidemiological studies suggest CBD has powerful anti-anxiety properties. Administered acutely ("as needed"), it appears safe, well-tolerated, and may be beneficial to treat a number of anxiety-related disorders, including:

- Panic disorder
- Obsessive Compulsive Disorder (OCD)
- Social phobia
- Post-Traumatic Stress Disorder (PTSD)
- Generalized Anxiety Disorder (GAD)
- Mild to moderate depression

CBD exerts several actions in the brain that explain why it could be effective in treating anxiety. Before we dive in, it's important to note that most research describing how CBD works is preclinical and based on animal studies. As the saying goes, "mice are not men" — and, results from animal studies don't always neatly transfer to human therapies. However, preclinical studies provide insights that move us in the right direction:

5-HT1A agonist: 5-HT1A is a subtype of the serotonin receptor, which is important because anxiety and depression can sometimes be treated with medications that target the serotonin system. This is why drug companies developed selective serotonin reuptake inhibitors (SSRIs) like Prozac and Zoloft. SSRIs work by blocking reabsorption of serotonin in the brain, which increases availability of serotonin in the synaptic space. This helps brain cells transmit more serotonin signals, which can reduce anxiety and boost mood in certain cases (although the full biological basis for this is more complicated and not fully understood).

Hippocampal neurogenesis: The hippocampus is a major brain area, and plays a critical role in a variety of brain functions. It's most famous for its role in memory formation and cognition. Brain scans of patients suffering from depression or anxiety often show a smaller hippocampus, and successful treatment of depression is associated with the birth of new neurons (neurogenesis) in the hippocampus.

An animal study using mice found repeated administration of CBD may help the hippocampus regenerate neurons, which could be useful for treating anxiety or depression. Research shows both SSRIs and CBD may promote neurogenesis. This is significant, because evidence suggests that severely impaired neuronal plasticity may influence suicidal behavior. Future research comparing CBD and SSRIs effect on neurogenesis could open up promising new avenues in how we understand depression and how to most effectively treat it.

Building on the foundation of animal studies, human studies are starting to provide evidence to demonstrate that CBD can improve many commonly reported anxiety-disorder symptoms, including acute stress and anxiety.

Human Studies Show How CBD Reduces Anxiety

Brazilian researchers conducted a small double-blind study of patients afflicted with generalized social anxiety. After consuming CBD, participants reported a significant decrease in anxiety. Researchers validated patients' subjective reports by performing brain scans showing cerebral blood flow patterns consistent with an anti-anxiety effect.

In another small study, researchers had patients suffering from Social Anxiety Disorder perform a simulated public speaking test. Participants reported significantly less anxiety, findings supported by objective anxiety indicators like heart rate and blood pressure.

Researchers concluded, "[CBD] significantly reduced anxiety, cognitive impairment, and discomfort in their speech performance," whereas the placebo group experienced "higher anxiety, cognitive impairment, [and] discomfort."

Evidence from animal studies have begun to characterize the details of how CBD acts in the brain, and human studies of patients with and without anxiety disorders are starting to validate CBD's efficacy as an anti-anxiety treatment. Given the huge social and financial costs of anxiety disorders in the U.S., CBD has the potential to play a significant role in treating a myriad of anxiety-related disorders.

While more research, including large randomized-control trials (RCTs), is clearly warranted to examine the long-term effects and potential for CBD, its demonstrated efficacy and highly favorable safety profile (particularly when compared to currently available drugs) make it a viable alternative or adjunct to currently available pharmaceuticals.

CHAPTER TWO

Healing with Hemp Oil: Your Ultimate Guide to CBD Oil

Perhaps you have heard of the many CBD hemp oil benefits – addressing physical discomfort, emotional homeostasis, supporting a good night's sleep and simply overall wellbeing. But then what? Even though the use of CBD hemp oil as a dietary supplement is relatively new on the market, there are many companies selling products that vary widely in terms of production and effectiveness. It can feel overwhelming to know what to look for when wanting to try a daily dosage for yourself.

In this ultimate CBD buying guide, we will talk with experts about the two most important things needed to experience the maximum CBD hemp oil benefits: the right genetic strain of a hemp plant for the best farming practices and a proven, effective lab production process. Without the right plant, there are no benefits. Without the right processing method, even the best plant won't help you achieve optimum health.

Ready to learn about what it takes to create the CBD hemp oil benefits you seek? Let's start at the beginning:

The Right Seeds

A seed is a seed, right? Wrong. So much of the hemp that is used to make CBD hemp oil today is low-grade, industrial hemp grown in factory farms in Europe, China and Canada. Because the plants are grown for a wide variety of uses – hemp is also used to produce cooking oil, clothing, non-dairy milk, rope and many other items – the seeds are not genetically screened for their therapeutic value. The plants are shipped in bulk to a facility for production, but the consumer can never really be sure what seed it came from.

"If you can't track your product easily back to the originating plant, then you may have cause to be concerned," said Dean Pinault, the farm operations manager at Functional Remedies. "We take a lot of pride in our farming practices."

At Functional Remedies, the small growing team uses a proprietary hemp plant that yields the highest CBD and low THC content, along with the broadest spectrum of other cannabinoids and terpenes. They are working to develop even better hemp strains with higher levels of CBD and other nutritional components as well.

Let's break that down: Low THC content means that the hemp plant contains less than 0.3 percent of the psychotropic component that makes someone "high." A high CBD content means that the plant is grown specifically for the therapeutic compounds that make the hemp oil extract so powerful.

Organic Farming

Of course, you can have the best seeds but poor farming methods. Many farms grow their hemp with massive amounts of chemicals to fight the weeds, but that results in chemically laced plants. For the four years that Functional Remedies has been growing, they've used cover crops like winter rye and good, old-fashioned hoes to address the weeds on the 65 acres they farm, Pinault said.

"Our practice are really important, because it all ties into basically having a healthy, organic soil and a healthy, organic plant, which gives you the best opportunity to maximize the specific genetics we have."

A new greenhouse and warehouse are currently under construction to meet the growing demands for production. Each year, they begin in January to prepare the mother plants for cloning to maintain the 90 percent stability rate of the seed's genetic profile. The new plants are then carefully maintained until April, when it's time to plant. Harvest takes place usually around August or September.

"It's not cheap to farm organically." "But we want people to have more options to better their lives with."

Accountability at All Levels

Once the hemp is harvested – each year has produced up to 20 tons of high CBD, high cannabinoid flowering plants – the crops head from the farm in Pueblo, Colorado about three hours south to the production laboratory in Louisville, Colorado. This simple transportation process also sets Functional Remedies apart from companies that use industrial hemp, said Kai Metcalfe, the production lab director.

"Industrial help that is imported tends to be stalks and seeds, but most of the cannabinoids and the terpene is concentrated highly in the flower and a little in the leaves and the stalk." "If the extraction is coming from the seeds and the stalk, that's a solid point I would question. CBD is not concentrated in either of those places. It exists, but it would be a red flag for me as a consumer."

Metcalfe receives flowers, some leaves and some stem – but very little stalk – in 55-gallon buckets straight from the Pinault at the farm. The first step to accountability is leaving the fibrous stuff out of the production process, and oversight happens repeatedly at every phase.

Using the Entire Plant

Another big difference among companies is that many use an isolate rather than the entire plant. An isolate is created by using chemical or high-pressure solvents to break down the plant into a white power that is 98 percent CBD. That white powder is then mixed into an oil-based substance to create the hemp oil. Some companies will use an extraction process and then distill it further to get the remaining THC out, and some companies add terpenes (the aromatic portion of the cannabis plant that has been shown to have health benefits of its own) back in for a richer nutrient profile.

But Metcalfe says science shows a full-plant product to be superior.

"The idea is the sum of the parts is greater than the whole. When you get isolated CBD, the range of efficacy is pretty narrow." "You have to have a high-level dose, but then if you surpass that you do not get constant improvement. And some trials showed that increasing the serving size of isolated CBD did not increase its efficacy for very long. With a whole plant, there is a much greater chance of increasing the efficacy when you increase the serving size."

It's known as the "entourage effect." The synergy of all the different compounds found in a hemp plant work in tandem to produce the CBD hemp oil benefits sought by the consumer. This happens only in a full-spectrum product.

Next, the way companies turn the hemp plants into hemp oil vary dramatically. Often, there is a chemical extraction process used. Companies will use butane or carbon dioxide as they pump high-pressure gases throughout the plant matter to break it down into an extract. That's not the method Functional Remedies uses.

"Our goal isn't to break the plant matter down, because everything we need is on the surface of the plant," Metcalf said. "We're not breaking the plant down in any way to get the extra bitter compounds. We're going for the cannabinoids in the trichome on the outside."

Metcalfe's team uses what is known as a lipid infusion process to create the oils used in tinctures, capsules and salves. What they do is steep the plant almost like a tea in either coconut oil or MCT oil (depending on the end product, since coconut oil can solidify when room temperature drops) at a set temperature for a specific time and pressure. Then they strain the hemp and dilute it into the correct concentration.

"There's no risk of consuming butane, hexane or heptane." "Tons of companies use chemical solvents in botanical extractions, but you have to be so careful and meticulous to get all the solvents out. The FDA has acceptable levels of chemical solvents in products, but nobody would want to eat even two parts per million of butane. That sounds kind of gross."

By using the natural lipid infusion method, Functional Remedies is able to offer a product with cannabinoids and terpenes as well as chlorophyll, flavonoids and other beneficial compounds found in the entire plant, Metcalfe says.

Understanding the method used in the laboratory is perhaps the best research a consumer can do before purchasing a CBD hemp oil product.

Quality Control

Of course, we've all read about herbal supplements that, after tested, actually contain very little of the beneficial ingredients consumers are paying for. How can you know that the tincture, capsules or salve you are purchasing is actually what the company says it is? Beyond tracking the product from seed to oil, you can look at the company's quality control standards.

"We test at multiple stages, starting with the initial extraction to see the starting concentration and then we compare that with the specification sheets for every product we offer," Metcalfe said. "We test, dilute, and then we test again to get the level we're aiming for."

By constantly testing of the product before being offered as CBD hemp oil for sale, the technicians can be confident they have not miscalibrated either too much or too little. This is an extremely important step, as it just one difference between CBD hemp oil and medical marijuana.

Medicinal marijuana – while containing THC, so the user will feel a perhaps unwanted euphoria and behavioral modifications – is also processed less, which means the user may not have as much control as to the dosage. When using CBD hemp oil, it is recommended to start with a small dose to see the impacts it is having on your health and wellbeing before deciding to increase your dosage.

Methods of Delivery

Once a consumer is comfortable with the seed genetics, farming practices, laboratory processes and quality control, it's time to decide the best way to consume CBD hemp oil as part of a daily herbal supplement treatment.

CBD hemp oil is not smoked. It is not vaped. It is digested so that the cannabinoids can interact with the receptors in your body.

"Hemp seed oil that you find in the supermarket and hemp milk, those are not sources of CBD," Metcalfe said. "Hemp seeds and hemp hearts that you find in the store, those are not necessarily a source of CBD. That's not where the compound is found."

That's what makes CBD hemp oil produced by companies like Functional Remedies different. The three main methods of delivery are:

    Tincture

    Capsule

    Salve

To decide which is best, take age, wellness goal and desired serving size into account. A tincture can be added to meals or tea, while a capsule can be taken at night like a multivitamin. A salve is ideal when there is a specific spot of physical discomfort or if a consumer has trouble swallowing.

With each method, you should feel as confident in the product as those who help to produce it.

"We have pride and love in what we do," Pinault said. "We take our time to get things done right. We always have the consumer's best interest at heart. We love what we do, and we do it in the right and proper manner."

CBD OIL (PLUS SIDE EFFECTS)

Cannabidiol is a popular natural remedy used for many common ailments.

Tetrahydrocannabinol (THC) is the main psychoactive cannabinoid found in cannabis, and causes the sensation of getting "high" that's often associated with marijuana. However, unlike THC, CBD is not psychoactive.

This quality makes CBD an appealing option for those who are looking for relief from pain and other symptoms without the mind-altering effects of marijuana or certain pharmaceutical drugs.

CBD oil is made by extracting CBD from the cannabis plant, then diluting it with a carrier oil like coconut or hemp seed oil.

It's gaining momentum in the health and wellness world, with some scientific studies confirming it may help treat a variety of ailments like chronic pain and anxiety.

Here are seven health benefits of CBD oil that are backed by scientific evidence.

1. Can Relieve Pain

Marijuana has been used to treat pain as far back as 2900 B.C.

More recently, scientists have discovered that certain components of marijuana, including CBD, are responsible for its pain-relieving effects.

The human body contains a specialized system called the endocannabinoid system (ECS), which is involved in regulating a variety of functions including sleep, appetite, pain and immune system response.

The body produces endocannabinoids, which are neurotransmitters that bind to cannabinoid receptors in your nervous system.

Studies have shown that CBD may help reduce chronic pain by impacting endocannabinoid receptor activity, reducing inflammation and interacting with neurotransmitters.

For example, one study in rats found that CBD injections reduced pain response to surgical incision, while another rat study found that oral CBD treatment significantly reduced sciatic nerve pain and inflammation.

Several human studies have found that a combination of CBD and THC is effective in treating pain related to multiple sclerosis and arthritis.

An oral spray called Sativex, which is a combination of THC and CBD, is approved in several countries to treat pain related to multiple sclerosis.

In a study of 47 people with multiple sclerosis, those treated with Sativex for one month experienced a significant improvement in pain, walking and muscle spasms, compared to the placebo group.

Another study found that Sativex significantly improved pain during movement, pain at rest and sleep quality in 58 people with rheumatoid arthritis.

2. Could Reduce Anxiety and Depression

Anxiety and depression are common mental health disorders that can have devastating impacts on health and well-being.

According to the World Health Organization, depression is the single largest contributor to disability worldwide, while anxiety disorders are ranked sixth.

Anxiety and depression are usually treated with pharmaceutical drugs, which can cause a number of side effects including drowsiness, agitation, insomnia, sexual dysfunction and headache.

What's more, medications like benzodiazepines can be addictive and may lead to substance abuse.

CBD oil has shown promise as a treatment for both depression and anxiety, leading many who live with these disorders to become interested in this natural approach.

In one study, 24 people with social anxiety disorder received either 600 mg of CBD or a placebo before a public speaking test.

The group that received the CBD had significantly less anxiety, cognitive impairment and discomfort in their speech performance, compared to the placebo group.

CBD oil has even been used to safely treat insomnia and anxiety in children with post-traumatic stress disorder.

CBD has also shown antidepressant-like effects in several animal studies.

These qualities are linked to CBD's ability to act on the brain's receptors for serotonin, a neurotransmitter that regulates mood and social behavior.

3. Can Alleviate Cancer-Related Symptoms

CBD may help reduce symptoms related to cancer and side effects related to cancer treatment, like nausea, vomiting and pain.

One study looked at the effects of CBD and THC in 177 people with cancer-related pain who did not experience relief from pain medication.

Those treated with an extract containing both compounds experienced a significant reduction in pain compared to those who received only THC extract.

CBD may also help reduce chemotherapy-induced nausea and vomiting, which are among the most common chemotherapy-related side effects for those with cancer.

Though there are drugs that help with these distressing symptoms, they are sometimes ineffective, leading some people to seek alternatives.

A study of 16 people undergoing chemotherapy found that a one-to-one combination of CBD and THC administered via mouth spray reduced chemotherapy-related nausea and vomiting better than standard treatment alone.

Some test-tube and animal studies have even shown that CBD may have anticancer properties. For example, one test-tube study found that concentrated CBD induced cell death in human breast cancer cells.

Another study showed that CBD inhibited the spread of aggressive breast cancer cells in mice.

However, these are test-tube and animal studies, so they can only suggest what might work in people. More studies in humans are needed before conclusions can be made.

4. May Reduce Acne

Acne is a common skin condition that affects more than 9% of the population.

It is thought to be caused by a number of factors, including genetics, bacteria, underlying inflammation and the overproduction of sebum, an oily secretion made by sebaceous glands in the skin.

Based on recent scientific studies, CBD oil may help treat acne due to its anti-inflammatory properties and ability to reduce sebum production.

One test-tube study found that CBD oil prevented sebaceous gland cells from secreting excessive sebum, exerted anti-inflammatory actions and prevented the activation of "pro-acne" agents like inflammatory cytokines.

Another study had similar findings, concluding that CBD may be an efficient and safe way to treat acne, thanks in part to its remarkable anti-inflammatory ualities.

Though these results are promising, human studies exploring the effects of CBD on acne are needed.

5. Might Have Neuroprotective Properties

Researchers believe that CBD's ability to act on the endocannabinoid system and other brain signaling systems may provide benefits for those with neurological disorders.

In fact, one of the most studied uses for CBD is in treating neurological disorders like epilepsy and multiple sclerosis. Though research in this area is still relatively new, several studies have shown promising results.

Sativex, an oral spray consisting of CBD and THC, has been proven to be a safe and effective way to reduce muscle spasticity in people with multiple sclerosis.

One study found that Sativex reduced spasms in 75% of 276 people with multiple sclerosis who were experiencing muscle spasticity that was resistant to medications.

Another study gave 214 people with severe epilepsy 0.9–2.3 grams of CBD oil per pound (2–5 g/kg) of body weight. Their seizures reduced by a median of 36.5%.

One more study found that CBD oil significantly reduced seizure activity in children with Dravet syndrome, a complex childhood epilepsy disorder, compared to a placebo.

However, it's important to note that some people in both these studies experienced adverse reactions associated with CBD treatment, such as convulsions, fever and diarrhea.

CBD has also been researched for its potential effectiveness in treating several other neurological diseases.

For example, several studies have shown that treatment with CBD improved quality of life and sleep quality for people with Parkinson's disease.

Additionally, animal and test-tube studies have shown that CBD may decrease inflammation and help prevent the neurodegeneration associated with Alzheimer's disease.

In one long-term study, researchers gave CBD to mice genetically predisposed to Alzheimer's disease, finding that it helped prevent cognitive decline.

6. Could Benefit Heart Health

Recent research has linked CBD with several benefits for the heart and circulatory system, including the ability to lower high blood pressure.

High blood pressure is linked to higher risks of a number of health conditions, including stroke, heart attack and metabolic syndrome.

Studies indicate that CBD may be a natural and effective treatment for high blood pressure.

One recent study treated 10 healthy men with one dose of 600 mg of CBD oil and found it reduced resting blood pressure, compared to a placebo.

The same study also gave the men stress tests that normally increase blood pressure. Interestingly, the single dose of CBD led the men to experience a smaller blood pressure increase than normal in response to these tests.

Researchers have suggested that the stress- and anxiety-reducing properties of CBD are responsible for its ability to help lower blood pressure.

Additionally, several animal studies have demonstrated that CBD may help reduce the inflammation and cell death associated with heart disease due to its powerful antioxidant and stress-reducing properties.

For example, one study found that treatment with CBD reduced oxidative stress and prevented heart damage in diabetic mice with heart disease.

7. Several Other Potential Benefits

CBD has been studied for its role in treating a number of health issues other than those outlined above.

Though more studies are needed, CBD is thought to provide the following health benefits:

Antipsychotic effects: Studies suggest that CBD may help people with schizophrenia and other mental disorders by reducing psychotic symptoms.

Substance abuse treatment: CBD has been shown to modify circuits in the brain related to drug addiction. In rats, CBD has been shown to reduce morphine dependence and heroin-seeking behavior.

Anti-tumor effects: In test-tube and animal studies, CBD has demonstrated anti-tumor effects. In animals, it has been shown to prevent the spread of breast, prostate, brain, colon and lung cancer.

Diabetes prevention: In diabetic mice, treatment with CBD reduced the incidence of diabetes by 56% and significantly reduced inflammation.

Are There Any Side Effects?

Though CBD is generally well tolerated and considered safe, it may cause adverse reactions in some people.

Side effects noted in studies include :

- Anxiety and depression
- Psychosis
- Nausea
- Vomiting
- Drowsiness
- Dry mouth
- Dizziness
- Diarrhea
- Changes in appetite

CBD is also known to interact with several medications. Before you start using CBD oil, discuss it with your doctor to ensure your safety and avoid potentially harmful interactions.

CBD oil has been studied for its potential role in treating many common health issues, including anxiety, depression, acne and heart disease. For those with cancer, it may even provide a natural alternative for pain and symptom relief. Research on the potential health benefits of CBD oil is ongoing, so new therapeutic uses for this natural remedy are sure to be discovered.

Though there is much to be learned about the efficacy and safety of CBD, results from recent studies suggest that CBD may provide a safe, powerful natural treatment for many health issues.

Advantages Of Cbd Help Oil

As CBD hemp oil becomes more popular in today's healthcare marketplace, many consumers are left wondering the differences and advantages between it and medical marijuana. After all, it's the same plant, right? Well, yes and no.

It's true that both therapeutic hemp oil and medical marijuana contain the most active cannabinoids found in the cannabis plant. Both have been used for years as natural ways to address to a wide host of physical, emotional and mental concerns. And by and large, both are safe.

But that's where the similarities end. The active ingredients in CBD hemp oil, CBD drops, CBD tincture and CBD salve have clear benefits over medical marijuana for today's modern consumer. Here is a closer look:

Relief, Not "High"

The active ingredient in CBD hemp oil is cannabidiol, which is extracted from the hemp plant. Yes, hemp is in the same plant family as marijuana, but hemp, by definition, contains less than 0.3% of THC, or tetrahydrocannabinol. THC is the chemical component that gets users "high," and growers take great care in increasing THC in marijuana plants. Hemp oil, conversely, is a non-psychoactive biological extract that is naturally processed from the hemp plant.

Without the psychotropic chemicals that cause a euphoric state, CBD hemp oil is appropriate for people of all ages. It is used to address unwanted health symptoms, not for recreation of any kind.

Hemp is a legal plant to grow. Unlike marijuana, which is grown for its high levels of THC in its flowers, hemp's stems and seeds are normally cultivated for everything from clothing to body lotion. When grown for the high-quality, therapeutic oils, the hemp plant is used for its CBD-rich flowers.

This is an important distinction, especially for professionals looking to reduce ailments, reduce stress or maintain health and homeostasis. If used at the recommended dosage, hemp oil is less likely of a concern during random drug tests (although this is something you should discuss with your employer). Mail delivery is not a cause for worry. CBD hemp oil is a natural, normal and legal product. You do not need a special medical marijuana card to purchase this product, just a desire to feel better.

Better for You

Using CBD in the form of a hemp oil tincture, hemp drops, hemp pills or even as a CBD topical salve is significantly healthier than smoking medical marijuana, which presents the risk of lung cancer. Even when eaten or vaped, medical marijuana's high THC content often has side effects like fast heart rate, slower coordination, bloodshot eyes and memory loss.

Hemp oil is different. Not only are there none of the negative health side effects with THC, CBD hemp oil has been used as a dietary supplement for many ailments. Customers say it positively impacts their mood, sleep, hormone homeostasis and pain management. CBD for sale is created using the whole plant rather than isolated compounds, offering users the comprehensive benefits that far outweigh those of medical marijuana.

Hemp and Inflammation Pain Relief

When it comes to inflammation pain relief, is hemp oil the answer? Discover what doctors and scientists are saying about this natural treatment of inflammation.

Before getting into a discussion on how hemp can help to alleviate inflammation we first need to distinguish the differences between hemp and marijuana. Both hemp and marijuana derive from the cannabis plant. The notable distinction is that the flowering marijuana plant has much higher levels of THC than the hemp plant. Tetrahydrocannabinol, or THC as it is commonly known, is the cannabinoid responsible for the psychoactive characteristics such as the sense of relaxation and euphoric high. Marijuana contains anywhere from .5 to 30% THC.

CBD Web classifies a hemp plant as containing less than .3% of THC. There are species of hemp plants that are grown and cultivated specifically for industrial purposes, such as clothing and textiles, but there are also varieties that contain significant amounts of CBD – another potent cannabinoid without the psychoactive effects but impressive healing properties. In any cannabis plant, there are over 450 substances, and only three of the substances are responsible for the "stoned" feeling.

What is inflammation?

The word inflammation is derived from the Latin word inflammatio, which translates to, "setting on fire." Inflammation in and of itself is not a bad thing. It is the body's normal response in repairing cells damaged by injury, infection, or allergic reaction. This type of inflammation is referred to as acute inflammation. The four classic symptoms experienced are redness, swelling, pain, and loss of function. Acute inflammation is usually in a localized area of the body, and the symptoms can be relieved with a cold press and topical inflammation cream. The inflammation will reduce as the body heals.

Chronic inflammation is associated with inflammatory disorders. These disorders are a result of a compromised immune system. Some of the diseases and conditions in this category are:

Acne Vulgaris

Asthma

IBS and Crohn's disease

Celiac disease

Rheumatoid arthritis

Autoimmune disorders such as lupus and vasculitis

All of these chronic disorders can interfere with a person's quality of life. Furthermore, complications from these diseases can be fatal. Unfortunately, these conditions can be complicated to treat. Cortisone and steroids are commonly prescribed, but come with many side-effects such as nausea, constipation, skin eruptions and rashes, weight gain, and sleep disorders, to name a few. Even OTC pain relievers such as Ibuprofen and Naproxen can cause an allergic reaction and with overuse eventual liver damage.

Natural Remedies for Inflammation

fruits and vegetables

Diet and nutrition. Of course, what we put into our bodies on a daily basis significantly impacts our health. If laden with an inflammatory disorder or any health concern, our diet becomes even more important. Our dietary habits are the first thing we should consider when thinking about natural remedies for inflammation. According to nutritionists, an individual with an inflammatory disorder or autoimmune condition should consume a diet focusing on the following foods, with the foods at the top of the list eaten in the greatest quantities:

Vegetables – in all colors

Fruits – especially berries

Whole and cracked grains

Beans and legumes

Healthy fats or EFAs- walnuts, avocados, hemp seeds

Fish and seafood

Healthy proteins – eggs, yogurt (unsweetened), high-quality cheese

Herbs and spices

Red wine

Dark chocolate

When planning your diet, of course, keep in mind any food allergies.

Herbs and supplements. Some of the most recommended herbs with properties that alleviate inflammation are:

Turmeric

Ginger

- St. John's Wort
- Oregano
- Basil
- Lemongrass
- Dill
- Cannabis/hemp

Hemp root, specifically, carries a substance called "beta-caryophyllene." Beta-caryophyllene attaches itself to the C2 receptors in our cells and in doing so helps to control inflammation.

Essential oils for inflammation. Essential oils that have been used to relieve inflammation include:

- Oregano
- Nutmeg
- Lemongrass
- Peppermint
- Eucalyptus
- Cloves
- Rose

Essential oils are administered in the following forms:

Topically – They can be added to creams, lotions, oils, serums, and salves. They are also added to bath salts and bath oils.

Aromatherapy – You can use them with an infuser, soy-based essential oil candles, or scented cotton balls strategically placed.

Orally – You can add them sparingly to water or tea.

When using, essential oils remember that they are very potent. They should never be applied to the skin directly, burned without being diluted, or ingested directly. When ingesting, make sure you are using a high-grade organic oil. If you have any questions about safety concerns, check with a professional aromatherapist.

How Topicals Relieve Inflammation

Topical applications can be one of the safest and effective ways to relieve inflammation and the pain that comes along with it. Since nothing is entering the bloodstream, there is no worry of side effects like and upset stomach or euphoric highs. Topicals penetrate the skin and work on a cellular level. By penetrating the C2 receptor of the cell nucleus, they send a message to the DNA. This cellular process produces a protein which to turns off the production of arachidonic acid which in turn reduces inflammation.

CBD Oil and Arthritis Pain Relief

Arthritis is the leading cause of disability in the United States, affecting over 50 million Americans. The two most common types of arthritis are:

Rheumatoid arthritis (RA): A disease where a person's body attacks their joints, causing inflammation. It commonly affects the hands and feet and leads to painful, swollen, and stiff joints.

Osteoarthritis (OA): A degenerative disease that affects joint cartilage and bones, causing pain and stiffness. It often affects the hip, knee, and thumb joints.

Some studies on animals suggest that CBD could help to treat arthritis and relieve the inflammatory pain associated with it:

A 2011 study found that CBD helped to reduce inflammatory pain in rats by affecting the way pain receptors respond to stimuli.

A 2014 review noted that in animal studies to date, CBD had shown promise as an effective treatment for OA.

A 2016 study found that the topical application of CBD had the potential to relieve pain and inflammation associated with arthritis.

A 2017 study found that CBD might be a safe and useful treatment for OA joint pain.

However, to date, there is little scientific evidence to prove conclusively that CBD is an effective arthritis treatment for humans.

A 2006 study found that a cannabis-based mouth spray called Sativex helped to relieve arthritis pain. However, this medicine was made from cannabis plant extracts containing both CBD and THC.

While findings so far have been encouraging, more research is needed to say with certainty that CBD oil is an effective treatment for arthritis pain.

CBD oil and chronic pain

Cannabinoids, like CBD, attach themselves to specialized receptors in a person's brain and immune system.

One of these receptors, called a CB2 receptor, plays a role in the immune system by managing pain and inflammation.

Researchers believe that when CBD enters a person's body, it may attach to CB2 receptors. Alternatively, it may cause the body to produce natural cannabinoids that attach to the CB2 receptors.

Either way, scientists believe CBD affects the way these receptors respond to signals being sent to them, possibly helping reduce inflammation and pain.

CBD is available as an oil or powder that can be used to make cream or gel, which people can apply to the skin in areas affected by arthritis.

CBD may also be taken in capsule form or sprayed into the mouth. It is a good idea to speak to a doctor before using CBD oil. A person should also educate themselves about their local laws on CBD oil, as the use of cannabis products is not always legal.

Small-scale studies have found CBD oil to be well tolerated, but some people may experience mild side effects. These include:

- Tiredness and trouble sleeping
- Feeling irritable
- Nausea

Risks and considerations

The United States Food & Drug Administration (FDA) do not currently approve CBD oil as a medical treatment. It is legal in some states in the U.S., but not all. It is a good idea for a person to check the laws in their area before purchasing or taking CBD oil.

Some people may have an allergic reaction to CBD oil, so testing the oil on a small area of skin is recommended.

As with any alternative treatment, it is a good idea to speak to a doctor before trying CBD oil.

CBD oil shows promise as a treatment for arthritis pain. The way researchers believe it affects receptors in the brain and immune system means it may reduce inflammation and pain.

However, more research is needed before researchers can say with certainty that CBD oil is an effective treatment for arthritis pain.

CBD Oil for Pain Management: Natural, Safe Pain Relief that Actually Works

If so, you know that pain relief isn't a simple matter of taking a pill and being cured. Chronic pain is a struggle day in and day out. More or stronger doses of painkillers often seem to be the only option. Studies are showing that CBD oil has powerful pain relieving properties comparable to morphine for some forms of acute pain relief. But more than this, CBD also promotes healing within your body, targeting the root of the pain problem — inflammation.

Its most effective treatment? Pain management.

Before we go much further, let's do our recap of what CBD oil is, how it works, and why it is NOT the same thing as marijuana.

Cannabinoids influence your body's natural healing and pain responses by affecting your endocannabinoid system. The endocannabinoid system is a part of many of the processes that regulate appetite, mood, sleep, immune-responses, and, most significantly, pain sensation.

Fun Fact: Cannabis isn't the only plant that contains cannabinoids. Echinacea, cacao, black truffles, black pepper, and kava contain cannabinoids as well.

How is CBD Oil Different From Weed?

CBD is a component of cannabis that does not contain tetrahydrocannabinol (THC). It is THC only that produces the euphoric and psychoactive effect that we associate with weed.

THC, the component that makes you high, reacts with the CB1 receptors, most of which are located in the brain. CBD oil activates CB1 receptors, which is why you're able to take CBD oils without becoming high or experiencing the associated symptoms of being high.

Recap on CBD Oil

CBD does NOT produce a high or change your state of mind. While derived from the same family of plants, CBD oil does not contain a remotely sufficient amount THC to produce a high.

Part of the hype over CBD as a pain reliever is precisely the fact that it does not alter one's state of mind — unlike most pharmaceutical painkillers, including opioids.

CBD influences your body to use its natural endocannabinoid system more effectively. Most CBD oil is extracted from hemp or special strains of cannabis designed for medical use rather than recreational use.

CBD Oil for Pain Relief

Pain is a major symptom of many short and long-term illnesses. Arthritis, Multiple Sclerosis, neuropathy, Fibromyalgia, cancer — the list of medical ailments that cause acute or chronic pain is nearly endless. Combine with this with pain from injuries, such as back pain, and you'll realize that just about everyone over the age of 30 does or will struggle with pain.

Age is also a pretty important factor for pain. This study found that one in four elderly people suffered from chronic musculoskeletal pain of a disabling nature. These figures from Australia show up to half of older people suffer persistent pain, and up to 80% of nursing home residents.

Cannabinoids trigger an anti-inflammatory response in your system, killing pain and even helping your body heal.

Researchers have stated that, "Studies in experimental models of acute and chronic pain have demonstrated the efficacy of cannabinoid receptor agonists, even in neuropathic or inflammatory pain."

Why Not Choose Pharmaceutical Pain Medications?

Use of prescription pain medications has increased significantly in the last decade, with opioids and drugs containing the narcotic hydrocodone as the most commonly prescribed. Unfortunately, these drugs are frequently associated with health complications, drug addictions, and fatalities.

Pharmaceuticals vs. CBD Oil: Side Effects and Dangers

Acetaminophen, a reportedly 'safe' pain killer, is the cause of almost 80,000 visits to the emergency room each year, and its overuse is now considered the most common cause of liver failure in the country.

With the wide variety of painkillers comes an equally wide variety of possible side effects. The primary concerns include the following.

High risk of addiction

Muscle relaxation and lack of muscle control

Muscle spasms

Nausea, vomiting, and diarrhea due to drug interactions with opioid receptors in the digestive tract

Heart damage and other cardiovascular issues

Increased likelihood of heart attacks

Liver and kidney damage

Potential birth defects and developmental problems in newborns (if the mother was taking painkillers during pregnancy)

Alternatively, research shows surprisingly few side effects to CBD oil. In fact, it is this lack of side effects that makes CBD oil such a promising pain relief drug. CBD oil

CBD does not alter your state of mind. For those who require painkillers to get through the day, but must also hold down jobs, this is an enormous benefit. With CBD oil, you can be at work without being in pain, and without being doped up.

CBD is effective without becoming addictive.

CBD does not cause any long-term damage or side effects.

CBD's antioxidant and anti-inflammatory properties support and improve the health of the body as a whole, including its impact of specific areas of dysfunction.

But — as with everything in life — there are a few possible concerns. The primary concern is that CBD oil can reduce the effect of other prescription medications, so don't stop, start, or alter medications without first consulting your doctor.

The following mild side effects typically occur while establishing a correct dosage for your pain, but may occur at any point.

Sleepiness

Dizziness

Dry mouth

Low blood pressure

Pharmaceuticals vs. CBD Oil: Expense

CBD oil is a comparatively inexpensive option to pharmaceutical painkillers. Those who are lucky enough to have insurance coverage often also have high deductibles or no prescription coverage. This means that the cost of prescription painkillers is often an out-of-pocket expense — and the cost can be crushing.

Pharmaceutical painkillers can easily cost over $1 per pill. Sound small? For those taking numerous pills per dose, several times a day, this rapidly adds up to a hefty price tag. When recovering from a surgery or injury, these medicines are typically used for a couple of weeks or less. But for those struggling with chronic pain conditions, things get expensive fast.

CBD oil, on the other hand, is a more affordable option. More or less can be taken depending on the pain levels being experienced that day, and can be stopped and started as needed. Lighter or stronger doses are available as well.

Pharmaceuticals vs. CBD Oil: Be Mindful

It's apparent that CBD oil can offer people with chronic pain an alternative to dangerous, habit-forming medications, such as opioids. Just keep in mind that because the FDA doesn't approve CBD products, they are also not regulated for purity and dosage.

What this means to you is that you should be extra careful in finding a reputable, high-quality brand from people you trust. This might be our team at Apple Wellness, a local supplement store near you, a medical practitioner, chiropractor, or naturopath. Just do your research first.

People suffering from chronic pain frequently experience additional health issues related to pain. Some additional medical benefits of CBD oil include relief for the following common side effects of chronic pain:

Insomnia: CBD has gained recognition by many medical professionals as a mild, natural sleep aid. By stabilizing your bodies natural symptoms and reducing the 'alarm' hormones related to stress, anxiety, and pain, your body (and brain) are finally able to relax.

Depression: CBD oil benefits include mood-boosting properties. Those with mild depression related to pain or anxiety find increased outlook on life when taking CBD oil.

Anxiety: CBD oil works some powerful healing when it comes to anxiety and stress. Research shows CBD affects serotonin receptors in the brain, activating more neurons and stimulating neurogenesis (growth). When this occurs, the mood is improved, and anxiety and stress are reduced.

Appetite: Cannabis has been used to stimulate appetite for hundreds of years. Many people experiencing daily pain, and especially those fighting cancer, have found that small doses of CBD oil can trigger a natural hunger response, while also fighting nausea.

CBD oil affects us all a little differently.

Your first priority is to find a high-quality brand of CBD oil. Both brands have extremely high processing and manufacturing standards, which means that we're confident that we're buying pure, natural, and untainted CBD oil. This is important — thanks to recent legalization, there are 'knock-off' brands that are more focused on quick production than on ▢uality.

CBD Dosage for Pain Management and Health Issues

Think about coffee — some respond a lot to just a little, while other people can seem to drink a gallon without batting an eye. All of our bodies process in different ways.

Because of this, we recommend that when starting out with CBD oil, start small and start slow. Gradually increase until you feel the results. Keep in mind; it can sometimes take a couple of hours for CBD oil to kick in. You'll have to be patient — don't give up if you don't feel any results within the first few days.

Take your CBD oil with or without food, in water, or right under your tongue. Food can help you to metabolize more quickly, but it's not necessary. By placing CBD oil under your tongue, you'll also absorb the benefits quickly. Expect CBD oil to take an hour or two to take effect.

Here are some general guidelines on CBD dosage:

CBD Oil for General Health Supplementation and Prevention:

3 drops in the morning or evening (2-5 % CBD) or 1-3 mg CBD per dosage, two to three times per day.

CBD Oil for Mild to Moderate Pain, Digestive Problems, and Insomnia:

3 drops in the morning and 3 drops in the evening (2-5 % CBD) or 2-6 mg CBD per dosage.

CBD Oil for Anxiety, Stress, and Depression:

3 drops in the morning, 3 drops during the day and 3 drops in the evening (2-5 % CBD) or 3-10 mg CBD per dosage

CBD Oil Dosage for Moderate to Severe Pain:

3 drops in the morning and 3 drops in the evening, after a week 5 drops in the morning and 5 drops in the evening, after 14 days 5 drops in the morning, 5 drops during the day and 5 drops in the evening (5-8 % CBD) or 20 – 30 mg CBD per dosage.

CBD Oil for Chronic Pain or that related to Chemotherapy:

4 drops in the morning and 4 drops in the evening, after a week 5 drops in the morning and 5 drops in the evening, after 14 days increase the dose further (10-25 % CBD) or 20 – 40 mg CBD per dosage.

Please note, these are generally suggested doses ONLY. The appropriate doses will depend upon the CBD product you choose. We do not ever recommend starting, stopping, or altering medications, including CBD oil, without first consulting your naturopath or medical practitioner.

CHAPTER THREE

Hemp-based Alternative Pain Treatments

Hemp is derived from the cannabis plant and comes from the same species as marijuana. The main difference between hemp and marijuana is that marijuana contains from .5 to 30% tetrahydrocannabinol, or THC. THC is the property which gives marijuana its psychoactive properties, producing the stoned or high feeling. For a plant to be considered hemp it must contain less than .3% THC. Hemp contains hundreds of natural pain relief properties.

Like most holistic and alternative healthcare practices, hemp targets the cause of the pain – inflammation – and works to reduce it rather than just blocking the pain. Modern day conventional medicine, such as non-steroidal anti-inflammatory drugs (NSAIDs) and prescription narcotics, work by blocking COX1 and COX2 enzymes in the brain to relieve the pain.

Hemp and Inflammation

Hemp has ideal properties for reducing inflammation, which is key in reducing pain. Hemp is helpful in reducing inflammation in conditions where the inflammation is either acute or chronic.

Acute inflammation is the normal healing response of the body responding to an injury, infection, or allergic reaction. Acute inflammation is recognized by its classic symptoms: swelling, redness, loss of mobility, and pain.

Chronic inflammation is the result of inflammatory disorders. Most of these disorders are a result of a compromised immune system and can impact the ▢uality of life and sometimes longevity as well.

Whether you are nursing a broken toe or managing the pain and discomfort from an auto-immune disorder, hemp can provide healing nutrients and valuable cannabinoids which work on the cellular level to reduce pain and inflammation.

Condition Alleviated by Hemp

Below is just a sampling of the conditions where medicinal hemp is used to manage pain and inflammation:

• Arthritis – Hemp relieves pain and promotes better sleep.

• Autoimmune diseases – Inflammation is the cause of illness such as lupus, fibromyalgia, and vasculitis, making these disorders responsive to hemp treatment.

• Cancer – Hemp has shown encouraging results in alleviating the pain associated with various forms of cancer and research indicates it may even stifle cancer cells.

• Chronic pain – Hemp works at the cellular level to relieve chronic pain in the neck, shoulders and back.

• IBS or Crohn's Disease – Cannabis helps with pain and digestion.

• Migraines – Cannabinoids found in cannabis and hemp can contribute to reducing the inflammation which causes the pain of migraines.

• Multiple Sclerosis – In addition to relieving pain associated with MS, hemp may also reduce muscle spasms.

Alternative Treatments Using Hemp

The entire hemp plant can be used for nutritional or medicinal purposes.

- Topical. Topically, hemp is used in lotions, oils, serums and balms. It is used for anything from chapped lips to joint pain caused by arthritis. It has a pleasant nutty odor and provides instant relief when applied, but also works on the cellular level. Through the C1 and C2 receptors, a signal is sent through the DNA to turn off the protein that is producing the acid which causes pain and inflammation. Topical hemp is derived from root serum and the oil of hemp seeds.

- Ingested. Hemp root is commonly mixed into teas, powders, and tinctures. Hemp seeds can be also toasted or eaten raw. Hemp oil is often derived from hemp seed and can be used in dressings and dips. Excessive use of hemp oil for cooking should be avoided as it can cause digestive and absorption issues. The nutrition of consumed hemp is important since it guards against many of the condition that eventually lead to pain and inflammation.

Alternative Pain Treatments Enhanced by Hemp Usage

Hemp treatments are a natural companion to other holistic treatments to alleviate pain. Besides sharing a history dating back thousands of years with such disciplines as yoga, hypnosis, acupuncture, chiropractic, and massage therapy, hemp also offers relief with minimal adverse side-effects.

Acupuncture, in particular, works very well when combined with topical hemp. The medicinal use of hemp and acupuncture both date back over 6000 years and originate in ancient China. They function very similarly at the cellular level to relieve pain and inflammation, while acupuncture additionally works to align the meridians. Both healing methods gained recognition throughout the centuries, but suffered legality issues in the 1930s. Today, they are both recognized by the medical and alternative medical community for their benefits.

Chiropractors and massage therapist appreciate the healing quality of hemp products and how hemp oils blend well with other healing essential oils. The cellular action of hemp enhances both chiropractic and massage therapy treatments.

Holistic hemp treatments are chosen by many over traditional pain relief option because of the minimal risk of side effects. Those already on medications to prevent blood-clotting, however, should avoid ingesting hemp in any form. Of course, any questions regarding using hemp with other drugs should be addressed with your healthcare professional.

4 Ways CBD Oil Can Help Improve Your Life

Today, there is no shortage of medical solutions available to treat the issues that we as people commonly face, from anxiety to pain. Some of these solutions are highly addictive or untested. One solution that has been gaining popularity in recent years is CBD Oil. CBD Oil, or Cannabidiol Hemp Oil, is a compound found in the plant cannabis sativa, though most CBD Oils come from the hemp portion of that plant. CBD Oil has been proven to have significant medical benefits for those who use it. From improved sleep to minimizing anxiety, here are five ways that CBD oil can help improve your life.

Improved Sleep

Many people today suffer from insomnia. Causes include REM Behavior Disorder in Parkinson's patients or REM sleep abnormalities in sufferers of post-traumatic stress disorder. Studies have suggested that a small amount of CBD can increase your alertness while minimizing how tired you feel in a day. This not only helps your daily work but can help further regulate your sleep cycle, improving your sleep.

Minimizes Anxiety

Studies have shown that CBD oil could also have a positive impact on those suffering from anxiety. Anxiety is an umbrella term to cover a wide variety of disorders that are one of the most common in the United States, which can lead to a variety of other issues. While anxiety can be treated with prescription drugs, many people are wary of these options as they can come with a wide range of side effects and the possibility of addiction. CBD Oil is a natural treatment that has been shown to help minimize feelings of anxiety, improving the quality of life for many people. As an added bonus, it is possible to buy CBD oil online. This can help minimize certain types of anxiety even further.

Reduce Acne

Several studies have shown that CBD oils can work with the internal systems in the body to help minimize acne. While this is still a new idea, the driving force behind it is that since acne can be a result of inflammation and CBD Oil helps prevent inflammation, the two fit together very nicely.

Pain Relief

For years, people have used medical marijuana to help them control their pain. Recent studies, however, have shown that the CBD compound might be responsible for this pain relief. CBD Oil is also not going to cause a high or any other side effects. What it will do, studies show, is to work with the endocannabinoid system in your body to reduce inflammation and to change the way some neurotransmitters interact. This helps to provide pain relief. CBD Oil has also been used to treat epilepsy and seizures.

It is important to remember that, as with all medical treatments, you should consult a healthcare professional to help you decide what type of CBD oil and how much at a time is right for you. Using CBD oil has quite a few health advantages that can drastically improve your standard of living. Whether you are suffering from acne, anxiety, insomnia, or pain, CBD oil might be able to help you improve your life.

CBD Hemp Oil Helpful in Daily Life?

Cannabinoids that are commonly produced by the cannabis plant, mimic the natural cannabinoids produced by the human body. These molecules associate with our endocannabinoid system, influencing many vital aspects of our lives, including mood, appetite, pain, inflammation, the immune system, and the neurotic system.

There are more than some benefits of CBD hemp oil over cannabis oil and CBD determines to be better in many respects. You will find more information online than you will find anywhere else. You will also find great sources of the quality CBD oil to buy. The uses that many people do not know about are more than what follows.

1. Addiction Recovery: CBD has been used in trials to improve people quit smoking. One study showed a 40% reduction in a figure of cigarettes smoked in a day. The impressions of CBD on other habits are unclear at this point, but it is feasible that CBD would be helpful for addictions overall.

2 Acne Relief: It works with topical application and maintains the pores of the skin to have the proper balance of oils for clear skin.

3. Diabetes: Mysteriously but surely, CBD has an effect for helping with diabetes. It blocks the production of a certain cytokine that immortalizes diabetes. This helps to block autoimmune disease development and lessen spikes in blood sugar. Additionally, CBD decreases inflammation caused by diabetes-related health queries.

4. Pain Relief: This benefit is really well known, but would it surprise you if you acquired that CBD oil can be as effective as codeine for pain? It works better than narcotics and does not cause an addictive high.

5. Fibromyalgia: This ailment is real and very painful. The pain from fibromyalgia can become so severe that it is disabling. Studies have shown that patients respond well to CBD for pain and other signs.

6. PTSD: There are very rare useful treatments for post-traumatic stress disorder. This is with standard prescriptions, not natural products. People who have PTSD report that CBD treats their symptoms and improved sleep.

7. Schizophrenia: Copious studies have been performed for the effect of CBD on schizophrenia. It has been proven effective in many cases and is now being studied as a medical treatment.

7 Observations from Using Hemp Oil Every Day for Three Months

Some people who have suffered strokes, cancer, depression, anxiety and general aches and pains have reported positive effects after using CBD, and the NHS is reportedly doing research into the compound with plans to officially class it as a medicine.

Until that happens UK citizens are free to buy CBD in its various forms online, something I first did a few months back and have been grateful for ever since.

Here are some observations from taking CBD orally every day for three months to help combat anxiety and sleep issues.

1. Sleep was immediately improved.

Issues with sleep is one of the main reasons I first looked into using CBD and it immediately seemed to have the desired effect.

Falling asleep was easier, while waking up in the middle of the night became a rarity.

On top of that, my dreams would often feel more lucid, and remembering them in the morning was less of a problem.

2. Concentrating became easier.

A task that might normally cause stress no longer felt like a big deal, while the process of doing the task felt more enjoyable and seemed to come to an end much quicker.

3. Keeping in a positive state of mind wasn't something I had to think about.

4. Cigarette cravings were reduced

The Beckley Foundation is working on a study investigating whether CBD could help with quitting smoking, after some preliminary data from animal studies suggested that CBD may be beneficial.

As someone who has tried to give up smoking at various points with various methods, to no effect, this was appealing to me.

And after taking CBD in the morning it became normal for me to not crave a cigarette until the afternoon, as opposed to lighting up soon after leaving the house.

5. It can work for pains.

CBD isn't just available as an oil but also as creams and capsules.

"Mercy had been complaining of severe pains down one side of her body after undergoing surgery and, after buying her some, the CBD was so effective that it's now become part of her routine too – replacing traditional pain medication".

6. Your tolerance will soon increase

Like anything you use regularly, your body will soon get used to CBD.

7. People are very interested in CBD.

Three people I know – my mum, a neighbour and a friend – started using CBD in the time that I did, after hearing me talk positively about it.

Alongside the effects listed above, researchers also claim that CBD acts in many of the opposite ways to THC, the main psychoactive ingredient in cannabis, and can reduce many of the negative effects THC can cause.

Does CBD Hemp Oil Have Side Effects?

CBD hemp oil is generally well tolerated, and it is mostly considered to be safe. However, it may lead to adverse reactions in some people.

The World Health Organization (WHO) recently reported that no public health conditions are associated with using pure CBD oil, and it hasn't shown any potential for dependence or abuse.

That said, some people have experienced side effects, such as nausea, vomiting, diarrhea, dizziness, dry mouth, changes in appetite, and bloating.

CBD oil can also interact with certain medications, and some of these interactions have the potential of resulting in more severe side effects, such as depression.

It's also important to note that hemp oils (and the suppliers for the oils) can vary in ▢uality, purity, and effectiveness. That's why it's valuable to do your research and base your purchase decision on ▢uality rather than affordability.

Before you begin taking CBD hemp oil, talk with your doctor to make sure that it might be right for you. Once you choose an oil, start slowly by only taking a few drops until you see how your body reacts to it.

Best CBD Hemp Oils For Anxiety

Now that you know about its positive effects, here are 7 options for the best CBD hemp oils for anxiety.

1. Nature Driven Hemp Oil Extract

Nature Driven Hemp Oil Extract is effective for relieving pain and anxiety. It contains 100% natural ingredients.

This oil is dispensed directly under the tongue with the dropper that comes with the bottle. It has 250mg of CBD per serving and comes in a one-ounce bottle.

Users have reported that this CBD oil is fast-acting and it tastes good compared to other oils on the market. It does not contain a flavoring like some other oils do which some people prefer.

2. Potent Naturals Hemp Oil Drops

Potent Naturals was created to meet the demand for a reliable company that specializes in the sale of safe, effective, and natural supplements.

This company practices fair pricing and offers customer-oriented honest and efficient service. They strongly value building a long-term partnership with their customers and keep your satisfaction with their products their primary focus.

This hemp oil is packed with Omega 3 and 6 fatty acids and works as a natural anti-inflammatory.

This original, top-grade oil helps relieve stress and anxiety. Each bottle of this brand offers a month's supply of 30 drops per day.

In each serving, you will get 8.33mg of pure hemp oil. Users love the peppermint flavor of this oil because it tastes fresh and clean.

Potent Naturals makes their hemp oil in FDA-approved facilities in the USA, so users can be sure that they are getting a high-quality product.

3. Prism Naturals Hemp Oil

This great-tasting formula was designed from the ground up and is priced reasonably so it is accessible to many people.

Every ingredient in this product is natural, so you can be sure that you are ingesting high-quality ingredients.

This oil has a slight peppermint taste, which users like. Also, many have reported that this oil works quickly for the relief of anxiety.

Each one-ounce bottle contains a month's supply. Users can take between one and two doses each day, with each dose being about 3/4 of a dropper full.

This hemp oil is made in the United States in FDA-approved facilities.

4. Zatural Hemp Virgin Cannabis Hemp Oil

This therapeutic, cold-pressed hemp oil has valuable Omega-3 and Omega-6, which can both help the body metabolize fat.

It is also great for skin and hair health. Many people use this product in smoothies, salads, vegetables, or drizzled on toast.

This virgin hemp seed oil is used as an emulsifying agent for our hemp seed supplements. The manufacturing process of this cold-pressed oil allows the hemp seed oil to retain its unmatched natural nutritional value and light, grassy flavor.

Hemp is known to be the most balanced oil for nutrition and it is easily digested by the body. Because this oil is a low-temperature oil, it should not be heated or cooked.

Additionally, it must be stored in the refrigerator after it is opened because it has a short shelf-life if left at room temperature. Users notice great health effects after taking one tablespoon of this oil per day.

5. Serenity Hemp Oil

The company behind this product uses a high-end extraction process to ensure the quality and efficacy of their product.

One of the most frequent compliments the company gets is that users are able to use less of this oil than others and get better results because of its potency.

Each serving (30 drops) of this natural supplement contains 8.3mg of premium, high-quality hemp oil. It has a delicious orange flavor which masks the "earthy" taste that some people prefer to avoid.

This oil also contains Omega 3 and 6 fatty acids and works as a great anti-inflammatory. Each bottle is two ounces, which is a two-month supply.

It is made in an FDA-approved facility in the USA, so users can be sure that it uses high-quality ingredients.

6. NutraHealth Essentials Hemp Oil

This full spectrum oil introduces the full power of cannabis sativa to give users immediate pain relief and reduce symptoms of anxiety.

Users have found this 100% natural oil to be very helpful in managing stress and anxiety. This oil is organic and GMO-free, and unlike other products on the market, it does not contain artificial sugars or preservatives. This product is 100% natural hemp oil in its purest form.

NutraHealth Essentials Hemp Oil is made from cannabis sativa and is cold-pressed in the USA, resulting in the freshest and highest potency oil possible.

It is rich in Omega 3,6, and 9 fatty acids, which can improve circulation and cardiovascular health.

7. Pepperwood Organics Organic Raw Hemp Extract

Organic Raw Hemp Extract comes with a 90-day satisfaction guarantee. The bottle contains 300mg of hemp extract, which is 10mg per serving.

It has a cinna-mint flavor and is made from the entire hemp plant, including the stalks, leaves, and the flowers. This allows the oil to obtain all of the nutrients of the plant.

This oil is especially great for pain, anxiety, and stress relief. It is blended with pure, organic hemp seed oil to allow for optimum absorption and bioavailability.

This oil is also gluten-free, GMO-free, vegan, pesticide-free, herbicide-free, and Paleo approved.

CBD Hemp Oil and Animals

Also our animal friends can suffer every now and then from unpleasant sicknesses - chronic pain, post traumatic stress, inflammations, skin issues, excessive fur loss, and so on.

In order to support the veterinary treatment or improve the general ⬜uality of life of our fury friends, you may try to use CBD hemp oil as food supplement, eventually as a medicine.

CBD hemp oil and the endocannabinoid system

CBD hemp oil influences the endocannabinoid system, which is also to be found in the bodies of mammals, fishes and molluscs. CBD hemp oil reacts with the endocannabinoid system via CB1 and CB2 receptors and activates the whole system - that means CBD functions in the animal bodies exactly the same way as in the human body. CBD has most of all pain-relieving, anti-inflammatory and neuro-protective effect and can be also used to support the loss of appetite.

Dosing of CBD hemp oil

It is know that animals could be picky when it comes to the intake of medicine, therefore we recommend you to put a few drops of CBD hemp oil with animal´s food or even some treats.

The dosing of CBD hemp oil depends from the weight of the animal. When you use CBD hemp oil as a food supplement, it is recommended to start with 2% CBD hemp oil 1-2 times a day: 1 drop - smaller animals up to 10kg; bigger animals (more than 10kg) - 1-2 times a day: 2 drops.

Already after one week you should be able to see some improvement in the ☐uality of live or even treatment of non-complicated illnesses. You can also increase the recommended dosage if necessary.

If you would like to support the treatment of your pet, we recommend you to take highly concentrated CBD oil - such as 5% CBD hemp oil or 10% CBD hemp oil.

The dosage is again very individual, depending on the illness and weight of the animal.

CONCLUSION

CBD oil is derived from the hemp, or cannabis, plant. Cannabis has been around for thousands of years, and while there have been hundreds of uses, such as rope, food, and clothing, the primary use has been for medicine. Hopefully, this list has given you an idea of which is the best CBD hemp oil for anxiety that could work for you. Try one and see how it benefits your health and well-being. Be sure to check with your doctor before using any of these oils to ensure there are no potential interactions with any of your existing medications. All of our Wellness Consultants are trained on CBD oil benefits and uses and would be happy to help you find the best CBD oil for pain relief. CBD may help with anxiety or mental health issues. If you are healthy and want to stay that way, the oil will make sure you do by protecting every healthy cell in your body. By trying CBD hemp oil you have nothing to lose and so much to gain!

Please write a review on Amazon, it's will be really appreciate.

Thank you!

www.ingramcontent.com/pod-product-compliance
Lightning Source LLC
Chambersburg PA
CBHW070116230526

45472CB00004B/1282